The Thyroid Reboot

The
Thyroid
Reboot

Identify and Address
Your Top 10 Symptoms
in 30 Days

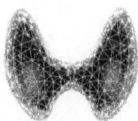

DR. JUSTIN MARCHEGIANI

HOUNDSTOOTH
PRESS

THE THYROID REBOOT
Identify and Address Your Top 10 Symptoms in 30 Days
First Edition

ISBN   978-1-5445-4763-3   *Hardcover*
      978-1-5445-4762-6   *Paperback*
      978-1-5445-4793-0   *Ebook*

Contents

Foreword

by **DR. DAN KALISH**

Founder of The Kalish Institute,
Author and Functional Medicine Practitioner

It is with immense pleasure that I write this foreword for Dr. Justin Marchegiani's outstanding book, *The Thyroid Reboot*. As a fellow practitioner in the field of functional medicine and the founder of The Kalish Institute, I have had the privilege of witnessing firsthand the dedication, passion, and expertise that Dr. Marchegiani brings to his work. In fact, he was one of my first functional medicine students, and it filled me with pride to see him excel in his career and contribute significantly to the field. This book is a testament to his unwavering commitment to helping people achieve optimal health and wellness by addressing the root causes of thyroid dysfunction, an area of expertise that he has pursued for many years.

Thyroid disorders have become increasingly prevalent in recent years and affect millions of individuals worldwide. The symptoms and consequences of these disorders can be debilitating and affect all aspects of a person's life. Unfortunately, conventional medicine often fails to provide practical solutions, leaving many patients in silence. We often find that thyroid treatments using medications exclusively fail to create the life-changing benefits we are all striving for.

The Thyroid Reboot offers a refreshing, holistic approach to understanding and treating thyroid-related issues. Drawing upon his years of clinical experience, extensive knowledge, and education in functional medicine, Dr. Marchegiani expertly guides readers through the intricacies of thyroid function and its impact on overall health. He provides invaluable insights into various factors that influence thyroid health, such as nutrition, stress management, and lifestyle choices, and empowers readers with practical solutions to restore balance and vitality.

Dr. Marchegiani's approach to thyroid health is both comprehensive and accessible. His passion for helping others shines through in his writing, making complex concepts easy to understand for readers from all walks of life. In this book, you will find personalized treatment plans, diagnostic guidance, and thyroid-friendly recipes that can be easily incorporated into your daily routines.

Having known Dr. Marchegiani from the very beginning of his journey in functional medicine, I can attest to his deep understanding of the human body and his unwavering dedication to his patients' well-being. *The Thyroid Reboot* is not only a reflection of his expertise but also a testament to his commitment to transforming lives by providing a path to improved health and wellness.

As you embark on your path to better thyroid health, I have no doubt that Dr. Marchegiani's *The Thyroid Reboot* will serve as a priceless resource, providing you with the knowledge, tools, and support you need to reclaim your health and live a vibrant, thriving life.

Functional Medicine Determines the Real Cause of Health Problems

I received my doctorate in chiropractic medicine, which is rooted in the vitalist philosophy that the body can heal itself; you just need to help remove the impediments to healing. Chiropractic medicine provided a solid foundation and dovetailed perfectly with functional medicine, which I spent most of my time studying and mastering, during and after school. Functional medicine focuses on the underlying root stressors of why someone may be sick and helps shift the body into a healing state.

Please do not confuse functional medicine with allopathic medicine, which is what your medical doctor is skilled in. Allopathic medicine uses drugs and surgery to treat and manage diseases. With functional medicine, we are not treating any diseases; we are working on supporting the underlying physical, chemical, and emotional stressors that create the environment for dis-ease to occur. I say "dis-ease" because in this state, a body is not at ease or in optimal health compared to a pathological disease state.

It was my own struggle with Hashimoto's thyroiditis that led me to dig deeply into how the body systems (System 1: Hormones [adrenal, thyroid, female/male hormones]; System 2: Gut and Immune; System 3: Detoxification and additional nutrient support) connect to each other. With this knowledge, I could help others *before* disease ravages their bodies, and *before* they end up on lifelong medications and need to have diseased organs or limbs cut from their bodies.

Yes, disease prevention is not glamorous, but despite this, getting to the root cause of what is driving the disease so that we can prevent suffering is my goal and the goal of functional medicine.

As a university student, I worked in the surgical field. Part of my job was to assist during surgeries with positioning patients, especially during diabetic limb amputation.

The surgeon would come in and tie off all leg arteries, for example, and remove the leg. I would hold the amputated leg, wrap it up, and take it to the morgue. The leg would still be warm as I did my job. Hundreds of limbs passed through my hands on the way to the morgue, and it disturbed me as I was confident the outcome could have been prevented.

This Had to Stop—It Was Ruining Lives!

I began to question myself: *How can we prevent this? How can we get to the root cause of this?* I asked the surgeons but got nowhere. It really wasn't their field. It really wasn't within their scope of knowledge or even in their minds. Most of them enjoyed the same vices (e.g., eating refined sugar, smoking, general lack of physical health, etc.) as much as the patients they treated. I realized there was a disconnect in conventional medicine regarding nutrition, diet, lifestyle, and getting to the root cause of their patients' diseases. Their focus was on finding the disease, cutting it out, and not preventing it.

An Ounce of Prevention
Is Worth a Pound of Cure

What do you do when your check-engine light comes on in your car? Do you cover the light with duct tape and pretend it's not there? Or maybe you reach under the dash and disconnect the wire? The best solution would be to take it to a mechanic. The mechanic can then find the source of the problem and fix it. Once the root cause is fixed, the warning light goes off.

Thyroid symptoms (fatigue, weight gain, hair loss, and dry skin) work the same way. The symptoms are your check-engine light. They aren't the problem—they're the signal that something is wrong. Just as you wouldn't carry around a roll of duct tape and slap it over your check-engine light, pharmaceutical drugs for thyroid symptoms may only mask them. Yet some people with significant thyroid issues may need natural thyroid medication to stabilize their thyroid (these are patients with very elevated TSH). This then gives you time to work with your functional medicine practitioner to ensure that the root causes of your thyroid imbalances are being addressed. It's always good to have your medical doctor rule out serious thyroid issues like cancer or a thyroid storm (severe elevation in thyroid hormones like Graves' disease), which tend to be rarer. This gives you confidence that nothing is being missed while working on the root causes.

What Is Hashimoto's Disease?

Years later, as I started dealing with my health and working through my own health challenges, I learned that I had an autoimmune condition called Hashimoto's thyroiditis. This is an autoimmune disease that affects the thyroid gland.

When you have an *autoimmune condition*, it simply means that your immune system is attacking your own body. In *Hashimoto's thyroiditis*, the immune system attacks the thyroid, and up to 90 percent of all thyroid issues are autoimmune in nature. I had suffered from the symptoms of severe adrenal stress for many years before I discovered this underlying smoldering fire called Hashimoto's that was residing in the background.

I diagnosed my own Hashimoto's thyroid condition while in doctoral school after finding mildly elevated thyroid antibodies in some of my blood work. *Antibodies* are produced by the immune system to fight off harmful substances like bacteria and viruses in the body, but in this case, those antibodies mistakenly saw my thyroid as harmful and were fighting it as if it were a dangerous foreign substance!

I was still consuming dairy and had nutritional deficiencies along with underlying infections that were driving my autoimmunity. Initially, this diagnosis motivated me to learn more about autoimmunity and the thyroid because I wanted to improve my health. I wanted to fix myself by getting to the root cause.

I then began to study the underlying connections that drive Hashimoto's. I learned about gluten and its connection to autoimmune diseases. I learned how infections can drive autoimmunity. I learned about stress and sleep. I learned about everything that could have contributed to my condition.

Thyroid Health Is Connected to Whole Body Health

After learning all I could about Hashimoto's, I turned my focus to the thyroid in general. I learned about the conversion of *thyroid hormones* (T4 to T3). I learned how to monitor thyroid function. I learned how the gut and gut permeability were connected to the thyroid, how the adrenals were connected, how food allergies like gluten were connected, how the liver and the body's detoxification system were connected, and how infections were connected. It was like a spiderweb. When one side of the web moved, the other side moved, too, just like the thyroid.

I also studied how the thyroid is impacted by toxins in our environment: blood sugar, diet, and lifestyle. I figured out what supplements were needed to help accelerate and nudge the thyroid and body toward healing.

The more I learned about the thyroid, the more obvious it became that many systems had to work together for optimal health. Thyroid function isn't just a one-man job; it's an orchestra, and if one instrument does its own thing or plays off-key, that beautiful music will turn into noise pretty fast.

As I dove into the field of functional medicine, I discovered that over twenty million Americans suffer from symptoms relating to *thyroid imbalances*. These symptoms include brain fog, sleep problems, depression, mood disturbances, constipation, cold hands, cold feet, thinning of the eyebrows, hair loss, lack of energy, etc.

Dysfunction in the three body systems (hormones, gut, detox, and mitochondria) can affect your thyroid directly and indirectly, causing symptoms to manifest. These body systems fall out of balance due to excess stress (physical, chemical, or emotional stress) in our lives, and our body loses the ability to adapt to them. So essentially, stress is the first domino to fall; body system imbalances are second, followed by outward symptoms. I call this the *S, S, S approach to healing*. When followed properly, it's a true road map to health. To help others attain optimal health, functional medicine was the ideal path encompassing a holistic philosophy, which I used to support my thyroid's healing and recovery.

The Difference between Functional Medicine and Conventional or Allopathic Medicine

Conventional medicine primarily treats these symptoms with medication. If you have a stomach issue, you are probably given a proton-pump inhibitor or an antidepressant. If you have a mood issue, it's Prozac or some other SSRI (antidepressant) medication. If you're fatigued, maybe some thyroid hormone or a methamphetamine stimulant will help.

On the other hand, functional medicine offers a filter or lens to look at patients and evaluate their symptoms. What is the root cause? What is the underlying issue? We don't want to treat and manage it; we want to eliminate and prevent it!

Imagine conventional and functional medicine as two separate tool belts. In conventional medicine, your doctor has only a hammer (the medication) in their tool belt. So for every thyroid issue the doctor sees, they pull out that hammer: "Here's your prescription for Synthroid, Levoxyl, or Levothroid, or some conventional thyroid medication." Thyroid medication may be necessary if your thyroid is damaged from a chronic autoimmune attack, but there is more to the story, as we address later in the book.

Here is the problem with this one-tool approach: What if the immune system, gut permeability, or a toxin is driving your thyroid issue? How does treating it with Synthroid, or synthetic thyroid medication, get to the root of the issue? It may play a role in stabilizing chronically elevated TSH and providing some symptom relief, but it doesn't fix the problem, and some may even feel worse. Hammers can be powerful tools, but there is often a better tool for the job.

In functional medicine, doctors and practitioners have many custom tools in their tool belts. These can include supplements, natural or bioidentical thyroid hormones, and specific lab testing to determine a person's thyroid pattern.

There are also the following interventions:

- Diet modifications (Paleo, low FODMAP, AIP, SCD, etc.)
- Blood sugar support
- Inflammation reduction

- Balance and support hormones (thyroid, male, female, and adrenal)
- Improve digestion and absorption
- Gut healing and gut permeability (leaky gut)
- Remove infections
- Support detoxification (of heavy metals, pesticides, mold, etc.)
- Enhance neurotransmitters and mitochondria
- Natural thyroid hormone support like Nature-Throid, WP thyroid, and other natural desiccated thyroid (NDT) glandulars

In functional medicine, the doctor will utilize every tool necessary to find and address the root cause (leaky gut, adrenal dysfunction, infections, etc.) contributing to the thyroid issue.

How Does Functional Medicine Address the Thyroid?

What makes functional medicine's approach to the thyroid so different, and why am I so passionate about it? It's because it has a very specific and unique approach to get to the root cause of each individual's thyroid issue. For one person, it may be simple: "Hey, we just need to work on your diet and adrenals and cut out gluten and grains."

For someone else, it may be, "You have some serious micronutrient deficiencies and chronic infections we need to address."

For yet another, it may be a combination of the two or three. My goal for each patient is to get to the root cause of the thyroid issue and customize a healing and preventive plan for that person.

Suppose we continue to look at where the root cause is coming from, eliminate the stressors, and treat the body systems that aren't functioning correctly. In that case, thyroid symptoms will eventually take care of themselves. We just have to make sure we do it holistically, and I will lay out the path to accomplishing this in *The Thyroid Reboot*.

What You Will Learn in This Book

In the book's first half, we will explore thyroid fundamentals:

- What is the thyroid gland?
- What does the thyroid do?
- What diet and lifestyle best supports the thyroid?

Next, we will address thyroid connections:

- The gut
- The adrenals
- Gluten, the liver, and detoxification
- Infection

Finally, we will iron out thyroid maintenance:

- Vitamins
- Minerals
- Herbs and supplements

At the end of the book, we will incorporate specific eating and lifestyle approaches that will help with any type of chronic inflammatory health challenge, including thyroid issues. I hope you will apply the action plan and utilize the recipes and meal plans included to fix your thyroid, increase your energy, improve your mood, and lose weight fast with *The Thyroid Reboot*.

This book is for informational purposes only. Please avoid self-diagnosing or self-treating. Please see a medical professional first and foremost to rule out any significant diseases. Next, see a functional medicine practitioner, and use this book in conjunction with the diagnosis, treatment, and advice provided by your practitioner. If at any point you need help during your journey to health, please see my resources section at the end of the book or at the end of each chapter.

This book contains affiliate links. If you purchase through these links, we may earn a commission at no extra cost to you. Our recommendations, including those from my family and me, are based on personal and patient experiences with these products.

1

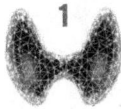

The Nuts and Bolts of the Thyroid

What Is the Thyroid?

THE THYROID GLAND SITS JUST BELOW YOUR ADAM'S apple or thyroid cartilage on the front of your neck. It is a butterfly-shaped gland that hugs your windpipe. You should be able to feel it easily just by running your fingers down the sides of your windpipe just below your Adam's apple or thyroid cartilage (tilting your head back slightly may help).

The thyroid gland resides and functions within the body's endocrine system. It works together with other glands (adrenal, sex, pituitary, etc.) to keep the body balanced and functioning optimally.

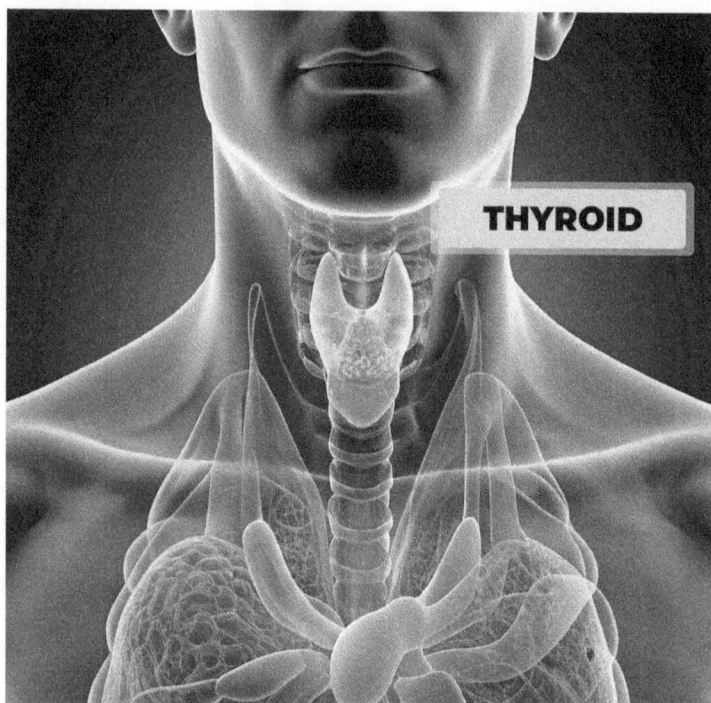

THYROID

What Does the Thyroid Do?

The main function of the thyroid gland is to serve as the center of metabolism in the body. *Metabolism* is the sum of all chemical reactions that occur within the body's cells; it converts the food you consume into energy. The thyroid gland produces hormones that help control and impact cellular metabolism.

You need thyroid hormone to metabolize other hormones as well, so the thyroid hormone is essential for life. If you don't have thyroid hormone or you start having lower amounts of thyroid hormone, you will start developing lots of unwanted symptoms, such as sleep issues, fatigue, and weight gain.

Think of your thyroid gland as your body's thermostat. If you turn the thermostat down low, it won't produce enough heat (thyroid hormone) to give you energy and keep you feeling comfortable. You'll start developing many thyroid symptoms, and your metabolism will suffer without the proper amount of hormone to control it.

How Does the Thyroid Work?

First, it's important to understand the hormone called *thyroid-stimulating hormone* (TSH). Conventional doctors will typically perform a TSH screening test when looking for thyroid issues. This is important because TSH is not a thyroid hormone as many people may think. It's actually a pituitary hormone. Since the pituitary is in the brain, TSH can also be considered a brain hormone. When testing for TSH, doctors are looking at how the brain responds to diagnose a thyroid issue. Clearly, testing the TSH isn't a direct indicator of thyroid dysfunction, but it can help pick up late-stage thyroid issues that may have been going on for years.

The thyroid gland produces a hormone called *thyroxine*, also called T4. Thyroxine is a *prohormone*, which means it's a precursor hormone that has less hormonal effect alone.[1] T4 gets converted to *triiodothyronine* (T3). Although T4 makes up most of your thyroid hormone, T3 is 300 percent to 400 percent more biologically active than T4. T3 is the most active thyroid hormone in the body; there is also an inactive version of T3 called *reverse T3* (RT3).

T4 primarily feeds back to the pituitary, telling TSH to go down as T4 goes up. T3 also feeds back to the pituitary.

Unfortunately, T4 is the primary hormone that most conventional doctors and endocrinologists test, along with TSH.

The following image is a good summary of how the thyroid works all the way from brain communication to the thyroid gland and peripheral conversion throughout the body.

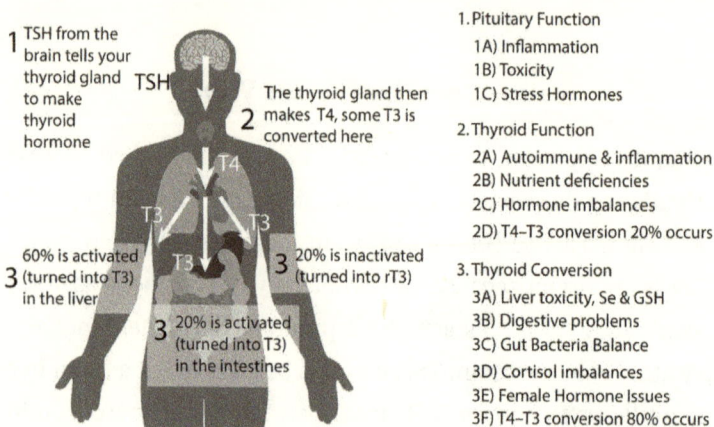

1 TSH from the brain tells your thyroid gland to make thyroid hormone

TSH

2 The thyroid gland then makes T4, some T3 is converted here

T4

T3

T3

3 60% is activated (turned into T3) in the liver

T3

3 20% is inactivated (turned into rT3)

3 20% is activated (turned into T3) in the intestines

1. Pituitary Function
   1A) Inflammation
   1B) Toxicity
   1C) Stress Hormones

2. Thyroid Function
   2A) Autoimmune & inflammation
   2B) Nutrient deficiencies
   2C) Hormone imbalances
   2D) T4–T3 conversion 20% occurs

3. Thyroid Conversion
   3A) Liver toxicity, Se & GSH
   3B) Digestive problems
   3C) Gut Bacteria Balance
   3D) Cortisol imbalances
   3E) Female Hormone Issues
   3F) T4–T3 conversion 80% occurs

Where T4–T3 Conversion Happens

Twenty percent of *T4-T3 conversion* happens right at the thyroid. The other 80 percent of the conversion happens *peripherally*, which means it happens in other parts of the body. Of that 80 percent, 60 percent happens in the liver, 20 percent happens in the gut, and the additional 20 percent is converted based on stress levels.[2]

Conversion in the Liver

With 60 percent of T4-T3 conversion happening in the liver, it's easy to see why healthy liver function has such an important connection to healthy thyroid function. If the liver is not functioning optimally, if you have blood sugar or detoxification issues, then you're going to have significant problems converting your thyroid hormone.[3]

Conversion in the Gut

With 20 percent of T4-T3 conversion happening in the gut, you need healthy gut bacteria for this to happen optimally. The sulfatase enzymes in the intestinal tract have the ability to activate T3 sulfate and T3 acetic acid. If you have dysbiosis (an imbalance of good and bad bacteria in the gut) from eating too much sugar or excessive antibiotic use, these habits will negatively affect how your body converts the thyroid hormone.[4]

Higher levels of the enzymes that help convert T4 to T3 (deiodinase enzymes—D1) also help with the reabsorption of the thyroid hormone from your bile and urine. Essentially, we can hold onto more of the thyroid hormone that is made when your gut bacterial balance is optimal.[5]

Conversion Based on Stress Levels

Additional percentages of the T4 hormone will also be converted based on your levels of stress. However, your stress level will cause T4 to convert to reverse T3 (inactive T3).

There are three kinds of stressors that impact this process: physical, chemical, and emotional (these three stressors make up the Triangle of Health, which we will discuss in a later chapter). Stressors cause the body to conserve its energy so it can focus on the stress. The more stress there is, the higher the percentage of T4 that is converted to reverse T3. The lower the stress, the higher the percentage of T4 is converted to healthy, active T3.

Think of reverse T3 as blanks in your metaphorical "metabolic gun." When you put blanks in your metabolic gun and fire it, nothing comes out, just some noise. The same thing happens with the thyroid when we put reverse T3 in the receptor site (proteins on the surface of cells that receive messages). The thyroid is not going to respond metabolically as if we had put free T3 in the receptor site.

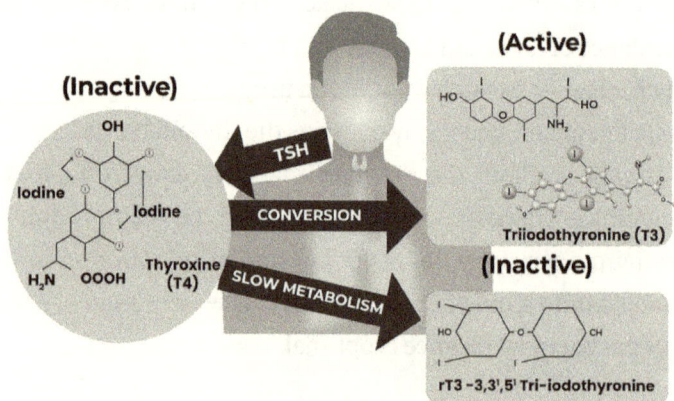

How T4-T3 Conversion Happens

Hormones have to bind to a cell's receptor site for a metabolic effect (an increase in cellular metabolism) to occur. This is true for any hormone—testosterone, progesterone, estrogen, and thyroid—to work.

Thyroid Hormone Binding versus Blocked

If the body is converting your T4 hormone to T3, that T3 can then bind to a receptor site on your cells, like a key in a lock (images A and B below), and it can produce a metabolic effect. On the surface, this might present itself as healthy hair, skin, nails, and gut function, for example.

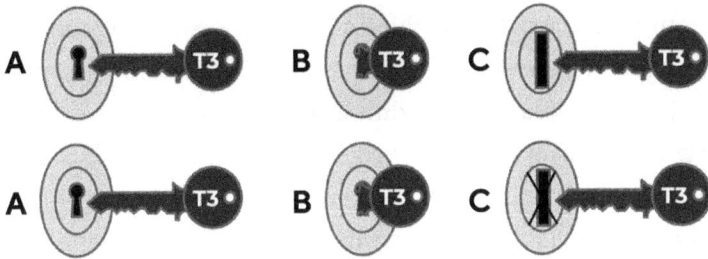

If the thyroid hormone is converting T4 to reverse T3 (the metabolic blanks), the body is telling you to slow down so it can prevent its metabolism from going too high. The key's inability to open the lock (image C above) serves as a representation of this. On the surface, this might present itself as fatigue, dry skin, constipation, and so on.

The Thyroid's Essential Ingredients

There are essential nutrients and elements that must be present to keep the thyroid healthy and functioning optimally. Iodine and selenium are the main ingredients, but just like with any good recipe, a little too much or not enough can ruin the whole dish, so let's explore these important elements.

Iodine

Iodine is the main essential element for creating thyroid hormones. The government's recommended daily allowance (RDA) is 150 mcg (micrograms) of iodine per day. When pregnant, your iodine needs go up to nearly 300 mcg. Inadequate iodine during pregnancy can lower your baby's IQ development, and it's the number one cause of preventable retardation, known as cretinism. As much as we think of iodine as being important for your thyroid, it is also very important for a healthy pregnancy.[6]

In the United States, iodine deficiency is rare because we regularly consume foods rich in iodine, including salmon, eggs, cow's milk, strawberries, and yogurt. Common table salt (iodized salt) is also fortified with iodine. Worldwide, however, one of the main causes of low thyroid function, or *hypothyroidism*, is iodine deficiency. Iodine deficiency is common in locations where nutrition is poor or where iodine is deficient in the soil, like in the goiter belt within the United States (the Rockies, the Great Lakes Basin, and Western New York).

According to the American Thyroid Association, Hashimoto's thyroiditis is the leading cause of hypothyroidism and it is linked to a heightened risk of developing thyroid nodules. Additionally, while rare in the United States, a lack of iodine in the diet can also lead to the formation of thyroid nodules.[7] One study following 2,941 people in a population where iodine was added to the food supply found the incidence of nodules decreased.[8]

On the flip side of the coin, excessive iodine intake can be a problem as well. Studies reported in the *Journal of Clinical Endocrinology and Metabolism* and others have shown high iodine intake can cause a *goiter* (a swelling of the thyroid gland).[9] For example, one study showed that in Hokkaido, Japan, where goiters are common, "the major cause of the endemic coastal goiter seems to be an excessive and long-standing intake of iodine from seaweed. In a few patients, restriction of seaweed induced a marked decrease in the size of the goiter."[10]

This shows there's a fine balance between not enough and too much iodine. This is why it's so important to work with your functional medicine practitioner to ensure you are achieving the proper balance. Self-diagnosing and supplementing with iodine could cause more damage than you are trying to prevent, and there are more factors to consider besides just iodine deficiency; selenium deficiency, which we will address in a moment, plays a key role here as well.

Iodide, Iodine, and Iodination

Iodide (I-) is essentially two molecules of iodine (I2) bound together. Your thyroid gland makes an enzyme called *peroxidase* that oxidizes the iodine, which means it loses an electron so it can bind to the amino acid *tyrosine* to make the thyroid hormone, T4. We commonly see this combined with *potassium iodide*, which is one of the more common iodine or iodide supplements used today. Some supplements, like Lugol's solution, will have a combination of iodide and iodine. Be very careful with Iodoral or Lugol's solution, as the iodine dosage is much higher than most—2 to 5 mg (milligrams) per drop with Lugol's. Make sure you are working with a trained practitioner when you are using higher doses of iodine. Supporting selenium and reducing thyroid antibodies and overall inflammation in the body and gut is always foundational before adding iodine at levels above the RDA into the mix.

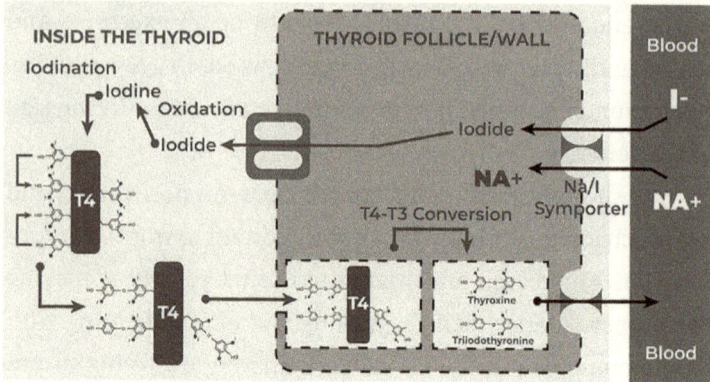

The conversion of iodide to iodine occurs through a process called *iodination* (see the previous image). This process involves the *sodium-iodide symporter* (the bridge from the bloodstream to the thyroid). This is where the nutrients from the blood come into the thyroid tissue to make thyroid hormones. *Pendrin* is the protein gatekeeper that helps with the transport of chloride and iodide into the thyroid cell.

Iodide is oxidized into iodine and then bound to the amino acid *tyrosine* to make the thyroid hormone T4, where it is then converted to the active thyroid hormone T3. Thyroid hormone (T4 or T3) gets its name because of the number of iodine molecules that are attached to it. (See the previous image.) There are four iodine molecules for T4 and three iodine molecules for T3.

The increased inflammation in the thyroid can affect the sodium-iodine symporter (NIS) system. This inflammation can also influence the way iodine is transported into the thyroid. That's why it's crucial to reduce inflammation and monitor thyroid antibodies before introducing higher doses of iodine or even any iodine initially.

Endocytosis is nothing more than the newly combined thyroid hormone filling up the reservoir of thyroid hormone in the thyroid follicle. It's like stopping off at the gas station to put gas back in your tank.

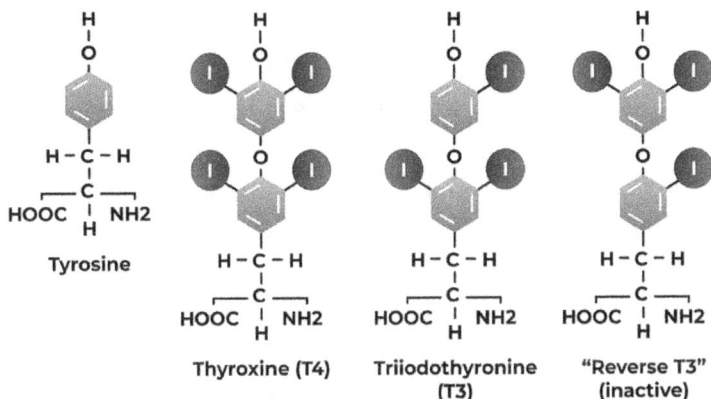

Tyrosine

Thyroxine (T4)

Triiodothyronine
(T3)

"Reverse T3"
(inactive)

Amino acids, especially tyrosine, are essential to making the thyroid hormone as well. That's why low-protein (like some vegan and vegetarian diets) and low-calorie diets can affect thyroid hormone production. Tyrosine ends up becoming a major building block for *thyroglobulin*.

It's a downward spiral effect: When iodine or iodide is lacking in the diet, iodination cannot occur effectively. When iodination is lacking, the amino acid tyrosine can't be bound to iodine to make thyroid hormone. This is how iodine deficiency can lead to hypothyroidism. Even if there is enough iodine but protein consumption is low, thyroid hormone production could still be impaired. Iodine deficiency isn't common in the USA unless you're malnourished from a low-calorie, processed-food diet and consume foods grown in iodine-deficient soils like the goiter belt area.

Thyroglobulin, Thyroid Peroxidase, and Hashimoto's

We have a compound called *thyroglobulin* that is inside the thyroid follicles and is primarily made up of tyrosine amino acids. The thyroid follicles are little berry-shaped structures throughout the thyroid gland. The thyroglobulin (tyrosine) gets converted into thyroid hormone via the iodination process mentioned above. Thyroglobulin (tyrosine) is bound to iodine to make the thyroid hormone.

Hashimoto's is an autoimmune thyroid condition where the immune system attacks the thyroid gland, resulting in lower thyroid function, or hypothyroidism, over time. In Hashimoto's disease, it's the thyroglobulin inside the thyroid follicle that is attacked, along with the enzyme that helps bind the thyroid hormone together. In practice, when antibodies are elevated, I clinically see TPO ab (thyroid peroxidase antibodies) elevated 70 percent of the time, while TG ab (antithyroglobulin) is elevated 30 percent of the time. Some people can go back and forth, like I personally have.

It's rarer, but seronegative Hashimoto's can occur about 10 percent of the time. Seronegative Hashimoto's is essentially someone presenting with autoimmune inflammation in the thyroid gland visible on ultrasound or needle biopsy without the peripheral antibodies coming back positive. It's possible the person's immune system may be weaker and can't quite mount a robust immune response, so the antibodies that are present are only locally available in the thyroid tissue and would avoid detection on a blood test.

This is another reason why I commonly assume that any patient I see with chronic low thyroid symptoms has autoimmunity to some degree, even without thyroid antibodies on a blood test being present.

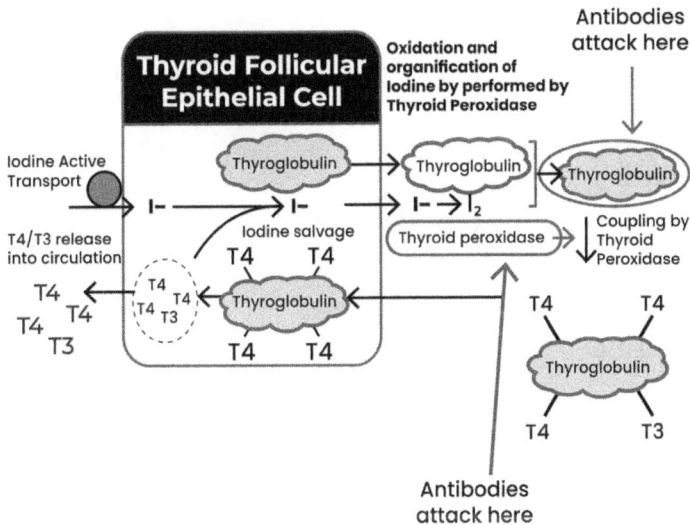

Selenium

Like iodine, the element *selenium* is also essential to your diet and thyroid function. It has anti-inflammatory benefits and can help decrease the antibodies that attack the thyroid gland. It has been shown that as little as 200 to 400 mcg of selenium per day can drop thyroid antibodies by 20 to 50 percent in just a few months. Selenium also plays an essential role in the deiodinase enzyme, which helps activate your thyroid hormone by converting T4 to T3.

One of the by-products of T4 metabolism is *hydrogen peroxide* (H_2O_2). Hydrogen peroxide can be inflammatory, and selenium helps remove one oxygen molecule from hydrogen peroxide, turning it into water (H_2O). The water is benign and safely removed unlike hydrogen peroxide.

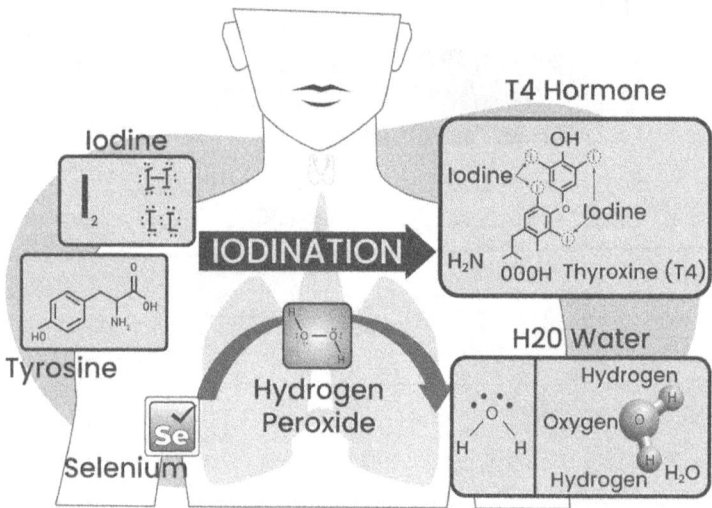

If a person supplements with iodine but has an unaddressed selenium deficiency, this can create a problem. When selenium isn't there to dampen the production of hydrogen peroxide, the inflammation accompanying it can potentially exacerbate an autoimmune thyroid attack.

Up to 90 percent of thyroid problems in the United States are actually due to autoimmunity, and this autoimmune attack is a hallmark of Hashimoto's thyroiditis.[11] This means the immune system is primarily behind most thyroid conditions and is not necessarily the fault of the thyroid alone.

So if we're just supplementing iodine to provide the raw material, that's good, but if we're taking abnormally high amounts of iodine and we're producing a high amount of hydrogen peroxide without having enough selenium to neutralize it to water (H_2O), the inflammation from the autoimmune condition will continue to occur. This is why it is so important to hold off on supplementing higher doses of iodine without a foundational treatment plan from your functional medicine practitioner.[12] If iodine is used supplementally, do not use more than the RDA amount of 150 mcg until your other micronutrients are dialed in first (magnesium, zinc, selenium, vitamin A, and CoQ10, to name a few).

There is a genetic predisposition that allows most autoimmune conditions to occur in the first place. As we move through the book, we will review the epigenetic triggers that you have control over that could help dampen and suppress potential autoimmunity from ever occurring.

The Bell Curve—How Much Iodine Is Too Much?

On one side of the fence, we have low thyroid function that is driven by inadequate amounts of iodine. If we have inadequate amounts of iodine, then we're not going to have enough iodine coming in to provide the building blocks to make thyroid hormones.

Insufficient iodine intake (most common worldwide), low levels of thyroid hormone, and thyroid autoimmune attacks can result in a goiter (when your thyroid swells). The TSH (the brain hormone) starts increasing when the thyroid hormone starts to drop or when there is insufficient iodine. It's like you're trying to talk to someone across the room when you're whispering, and that person can't hear you unless you increase the volume.[13]

It's the same thing when the pituitary and the brain (TSH) are talking to the thyroid. If the release of thyroid hormone (T4, T3) is too low, the TSH has to increase; it has to start to increase the volume until it gets a response. Without the iodine present as the building block to make the thyroid hormone or adequate levels of T4 or T3, the TSH will continue to increase, and the thyroid gland can start to swell. The swelling is a result of elevated TSH yelling at the thyroid gland to make more thyroid hormone; there is not enough hormone being made.

On the other side of the fence, in cultures that consume high amounts of iodine—such as excessive amounts of iodized salt, extra supplemental iodine, or seaweed like kelp or dulse—we can see an increase in Hashimoto's.[14] The extra iodine stimulates hydrogen peroxide (H_2O_2), and without the high levels of selenium being there to turn it into water (H_2O), the hydrogen peroxide can create inflammation. The inflammation from the thyroid attack can be enough to enlarge the thyroid to the point where a goiter or nodule may develop.

Our immune system responds by sending B cells to clean up the inflammation, and while that's happening, we're developing specific thyroid antibodies against your thyroid tissue as a result of the immune response. The two major antibodies that are increased during the autoimmune response are thyroglobulin (the thyroid protein inside the thyroid follicles) and thyroid peroxidase (an enzyme that helps make the thyroid hormone). The more this autoimmune response occurs, the more the thyroid tissue can become fibrotic, and scar tissue can actually develop. Eventually, the thyroid tissues become less functional, and they won't be able to do what they were designed to do, which is make the thyroid hormone. Imagine your thyroid as a three- to four-month reservoir for thyroid hormone. It holds thyroid hormone in little follicles that look like berries. When your immune system attacks your thyroid, it starts to pop each berry one by one. Each knife represents either thyroid peroxidase antibodies (TPO ab) or thyroglobulin antibodies (TG ab).[15]

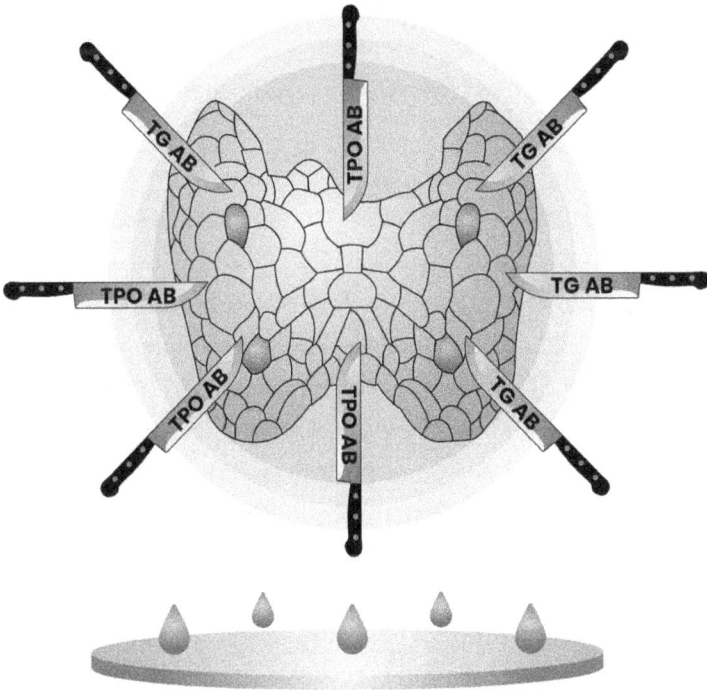

Pro tip: Low-level laser therapy (LLLT) has emerged as a promising approach for reducing thyroid inflammation in individuals with Hashimoto's thyroiditis. By applying low-dose laser light directly to the thyroid gland, LLLT can help decrease inflammation, improve thyroid function and even stimulate regeneration. This non-invasive treatment enhances cellular metabolism and reduces oxidative stress, factors that are often implicated in the autoimmune response of Hashimoto's. Early research suggests that LLLT may reduce the need for medication in some patients by improving thyroid gland health and reducing antibody levels associated with this condition. At the end of this chapter, we will include a reference for accessing a therapeutic-grade laser capable of providing these benefits.[16]

Higher levels of iodine were recommended based on previous survey data out of Japan showing iodine intake via seaweed as high as 13.5 to 45 mg per day. Many doctors said, "Well, if we are getting that much in food, let's try it via supplementation."

Over the last few decades, research has shown that iodine intake is extremely overestimated. The current estimated intake of iodine in Japan is around 1 to 3 mg per day, over ten times less than what it was thought to be originally. Based on this new data, I typically don't recommend supplementing more than the 1 mg range, especially with the understanding that hydrogen peroxide can be produced during the iodination process, which can increase autoimmune thyroid inflammation.[17]

It's always best to start at the RDA of 150 mcg and then work up only when thyroid inflammation is stable. It's important to work with a functional medicine clinician to ensure your thyroid and antibodies are not increasing during the process and that the other cofactors for the thyroid are present, like selenium, zinc, magnesium, and copper. Don't forget that a small percentage of the time, patients can have Hashimoto's without a positive blood test for elevated TPO and TG antibodies.

There are well-established doctors who hold differing views on iodine supplementation. For instance, Dr. Brownstein advocates for high levels of iodine supplementation, whereas Dr. Kharrazian recommends minimal to no iodine supplementation, and even advises against consuming iodine-rich foods like seaweed or iodized salt, especially for patients with Hashimoto's.[18] Both of these doctors have great clinical success, and the data in the peer-reviewed literature could be cherry-picked to support each side, as I showed above. My belief is that the truth probably lies somewhere in between, maybe a little different for each person. This is why you need a comprehensive functional medicine approach that goes far beyond just iodine supplements to optimize thyroid health.

Hashimoto's Thyroiditis

Hashimoto's thyroiditis is an autoimmune condition of the thyroid thought to be present in anywhere between 30 percent to 90 percent of hypothyroidism cases in the United States, depending on the study you read.[19] Japanese physician Hakaru

Hashimoto first noted Hashimoto's in 1912. He termed the disease *struma lymphomatosa*.[20]

There's a phenomenon known in Hashimoto's that may be active, and it's known as *molecular mimicry*, which basically means that the immune system sees the proteins of a foreign invader (e.g., bacteria or virus) looking similar to the proteins of the thyroid. This results in the immune system misidentifying and attacking invaders and its own thyroid tissue. *Autoimmune* means "immune to self"—the body essentially attacks itself.[21]

This is like the police putting out an APB for a black car that was seen near a recent robbery. You may happen to be driving by that area in a black car yourself and get pulled over accidentally. Just like the police pulled you over in a black car, the immune system similarly may attack other healthy tissues in the body.

Inflammation is a by-product of autoimmune conditions, degrading the function of the thyroid gland over time. When the immune system mistakenly attacks the body, inflammation occurs as a natural response. In the case of chronic thyroid inflammation, the output of the gland can be affected, leading to decreased hormone production of T4 and T3, as well as an increase in TSH as a result. Additionally, the presence of elevated levels of cytokines, interleukins, and other inflammatory compounds in the bloodstream can have an impact on lowering T3 hormone levels as well. TSH elevations can take quite a while to be at a threshold for a thyroid problem to be diagnosed. All the while, more inflammation due to autoimmunity is occurring.[22]

Research shows that when thyroid antibodies were elevated women were over two times more likely to have elevated

TSH levels.[23] Also, when TSH levels increased above 2.5, more patients with positive thyroid antibodies were seen.

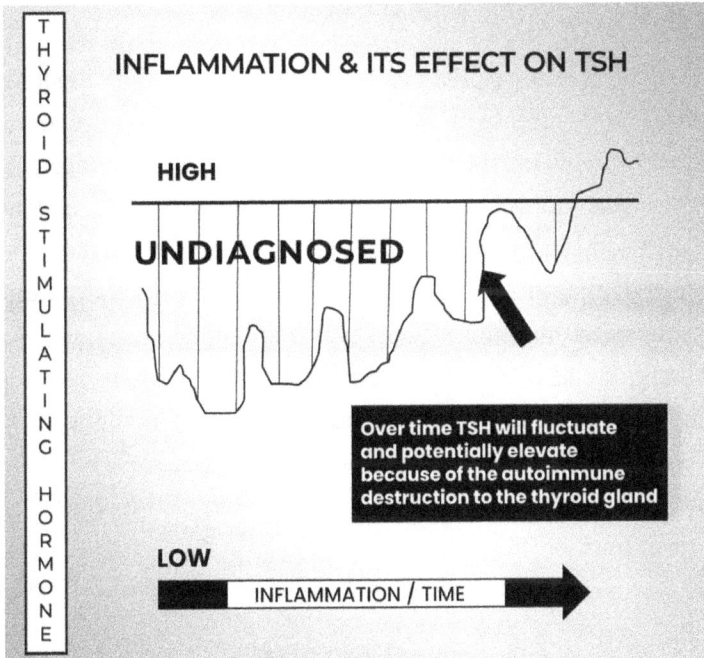

INFLAMMATION & ITS EFFECT ON TSH

THYROID STIMULATING HORMONE

HIGH

UNDIAGNOSED

Over time TSH will fluctuate and potentially elevate because of the autoimmune destruction to the thyroid gland

LOW

INFLAMMATION / TIME

I surmise that inflammation from the autoimmune attack is impacting the thyroid follicles from making optimal levels of thyroid hormone. Then the pituitary is responding by increasing TSH to compensate for the lack of thyroid hormone.

In Hashimoto's disease, the thyroid gland can become enlarged due to increasing inflammation and elevated TSH, and it can possibly become nodular as well.[24] Many root causes can exacerbate this, including the following. Chronically elevated TSH levels are also associated with a higher risk of thyroid cancer.[25]

- Nutritional imbalances (iodine, selenium, etc.)
- Gluten and grains
- Infections

According to a study, persistent thyroid inflammation and Hashimoto's disease can elevate the risk of thyroid cancer over time. Moreover, this risk extends beyond thyroid cancer to other types of cancer, such as breast, lung, digestive, urogenital, blood, and prolactinomas. The underlying mechanism causing inflammation in the thyroid can have a systemic effect on the entire immune system. There are numerous strategies we employ in this book to enhance thyroid function, including addressing dysglycemia and supporting vitamin D and glutathione levels, to name just a few. These measures not only improve your immune system but also have positive effects on preventing and combating cancer.[26]

Hypothyroidism

Hypothyroidism is the underproduction of thyroid hormone, typically followed by an elevation in TSH. The TSH is trying to scream down to the thyroid from the pituitary to make thyroid hormone. Symptoms such as weight gain, dry hair and skin, and fatigue are typically not alleviated by conventional thyroid medications such as Synthroid or Levoxyl. The good news is that addressing the root cause can alleviate these symptoms. The root causes of hypothyroidism can be traced to many sources, including the following:

- Hashimoto's thyroiditis

- Adrenal dysfunction
- Selenium deficiency
- Iodine deficiency
- Anemia (iron or B_{12})
- Infections
- Blood sugar swings
- Low stomach acid and enzyme production
- Lower calories or excessive fasting

Hyperthyroidism is the overproduction of thyroid hormone. Graves' disease, another autoimmune condition, is the main cause of it. In the United States, only about 1 percent of thyroid conditions are hyperthyroid, and out of that 1 percent of hyperthyroid cases, 80 percent of those cases are Graves' disease (autoimmune in nature).[27]

Graves' disease may present with the following symptoms: exophthalmos (eyeballs starting to bulge), excessive sweating, increased irritability, insomnia, weight loss, anxiety, diarrhea, shakiness, increased heart rate, and typically lower levels of TSH (which go lower when thyroid hormone goes higher).

If you're already taking thyroid hormone, that can cause the TSH to drop as well. Conventional doctors will run a TSH test when a patient is on a thyroid supplement or thyroid medication, and they may see an incredibly low TSH and think the patient has a hyperthyroid condition. Yet if they actually ran T4 and T3 tests, they would see that the thyroid hormone levels are perfect. So if someone's on thyroid medication, the TSH will be less reliable, but we typically shoot for a TSH between 0.5 and 2.5; 1.5 being ideal. It's very important that when looking at

TSH, you still look at all the other thyroid hormones, take into account where the patient feels best, and factor in their basal body temperature too.

GRAVES' DISEASE SYMPTOMS

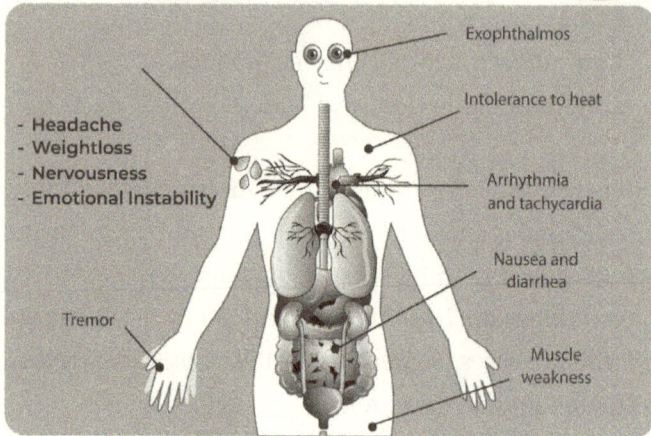

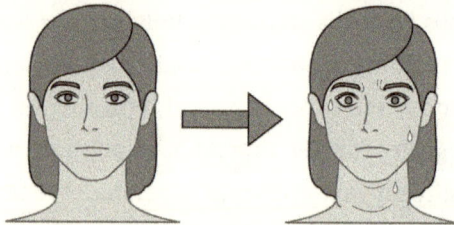

- Headache
- Weightloss
- Nervousness
- Emotional Instability

Exophthalmos

Intolerance to heat

Arrhythmia and tachycardia

Nausea and diarrhea

Tremor

Muscle weakness

If someone's not on thyroid hormone, the TSH can be more valuable at picking up Graves' disease, but we also have to look at the direct thyroid hormone levels instead of fully relying on the indirect brain hormone TSH.

To assess Graves', we would want to run the following tests: TSH, T4 free, T4 total, T3 free, T3 total, as well as specific antibodies that are the hallmark of Graves': thyrotropin receptor antibody (TRAb) and thyroid-stimulating immunoglobulins (TSI), which are types of TRAb. They attach to thyroid cell receptors, which typically serve as binding sites for thyroid-stimulating hormone (TSH). By doing so, TSI deceives the thyroid gland into expanding and generating an excess of thyroid hormone, ultimately resulting in hyperthyroidism.

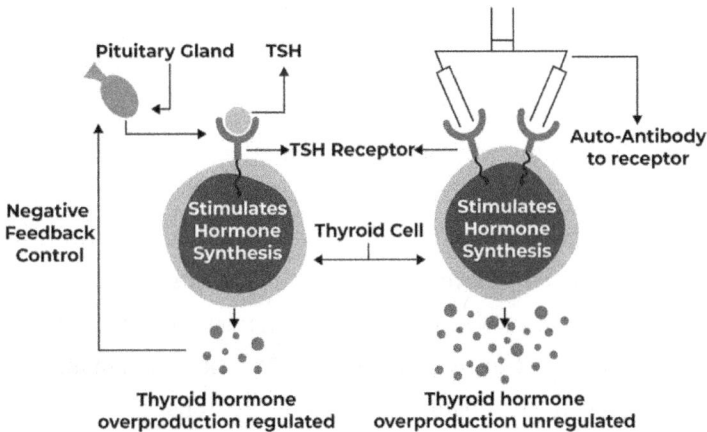

The biggest difference between Hashimoto's and Graves' disease is that Graves' is an autoimmune attack on the outside of the thyroid gland that stimulates more thyroid production (see above), while Hashimoto's is more of an internal autoimmune attack on the thyroid tissue (thyroid proteins and enzymes). Patients with Hashimoto's may present with Graves' or hyperthyroid-like symptoms because the autoimmunity condition can cause thyroid hormones to spill from the thyroid follicles during the autoimmune attack.

Our thyroid stores about three to four months' worth of thyroid hormone, so there are some reserves within the thyroid tissue.[28] This jump in hormone levels can feel like a hyperthyroid situation, like in Graves' disease. That's why you want to test all thyroid hormones and antibodies to make sure you know what you are dealing with.

If it's not Hashimoto's, we want to fully evaluate if it is Graves' because Graves' left untreated can cause heart damage or stroke and can be life threatening. If we are having hyperthyroid symptoms, we want to get the right test done to evaluate if Graves' disease is occurring. Once Graves' disease is diagnosed, depending on how advanced it is, we may be able to add natural strategies to cool the thyroid down before resorting to a more extreme approach, such as removing the thyroid or performing a radioactive thyroid ablation, which shuts down the thyroid using radioactive iodine. The sooner we catch it, the more conservative we can be in our strategy to control and manage it with nutrients, botanicals, diet, and lifestyle changes.

The typical medications recommended for Graves' are methimazole and propylthiouracil (PTU), which block thyroid hormone synthesis and thyroid hormone conversion (T4 to T3). Beta-blockers are also recommended to calm the heart rate and blood pressure caused by the elevated thyroid hormone. These medications may be necessary if there is an acute flare while you work on getting to the root cause with your functional medicine doctor. Always get Graves' ruled out by your medical doctor and try to hold off on the more extreme surgical and radiation options if medically possible.[29]

Goiter

A goiter is a swelling or abnormal enlargement of the thyroid gland. This condition can arise when the feedback loop to TSH is disrupted due to low levels of thyroid hormones, leading to increased TSH production by the pituitary gland.

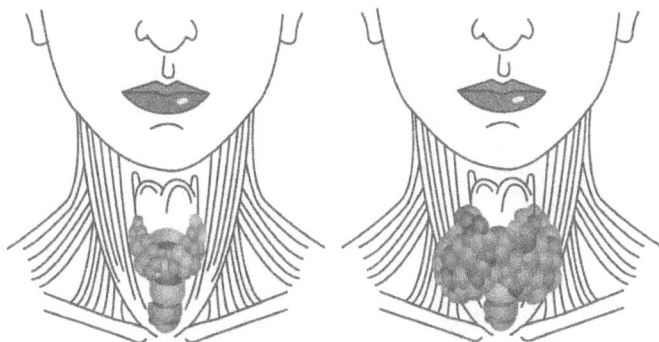

Several factors can drive the development of a goiter. Low iodine intake may result in inadequate building blocks for thyroid hormone production, leading to lower hormone levels. Increased inflammation from an autoimmune attack like in Graves' and Hashimoto's. Chronic stress can also dysregulate the hypothalamic-pituitary-thyroid (HPT) axis, further disrupting TSH levels, and contributing to thyroid swelling.

As shown in the Hokkaido, Japan, study in the iodine section of this chapter, too much iodine can also be a culprit in causing goiter.[30] This is why it is so important to work with your practitioner to find the ideal balance. I typically frown upon using megadoses of iodine, more than a few milligrams, for the thyroid unless you are working with a skilled functional medicine practitioner who is monitoring your thyroid closely.

Thyroid Patient Exam

During the patient's exam to assess the thyroid, the Triple-S Approach is a technique that can be used to thoroughly review your health status. The Triple-S Approach focuses on the following:

1. Assess All Lifestyle Stressors (the Triangle of Health—physical, chemical, and emotional stress)
2. Body Systems Assessment:
    a. System 1: Hormones (adrenal, thyroid, female/male hormones)
    b. System 2: Gut and Immune
    c. System 3: Detoxification and additional nutrient support)
3. Assess Symptoms (cold hands, cold feet, hair loss, eyebrow thinning, constipation, and low body temp)
4. Palpation of the thyroid to assess inflammation physically
5. Full thyroid hormone profile including thyroid antibodies; Graves' antibody only when TSH is very low, Graves' symptoms are present, and thyroid hormones are elevated
6. Thyroid ultrasound if no thyroid antibodies are present (it is thought that 10 percent of the population may have Hashimoto's and does not present with thyroid antibodies)

Stressors (the Triangle of Health)

Stressors come in three major forms, and these make up the Triangle of Health, which is a concept that shows the need for balance among all three stressors: emotional, physical, and chemical.

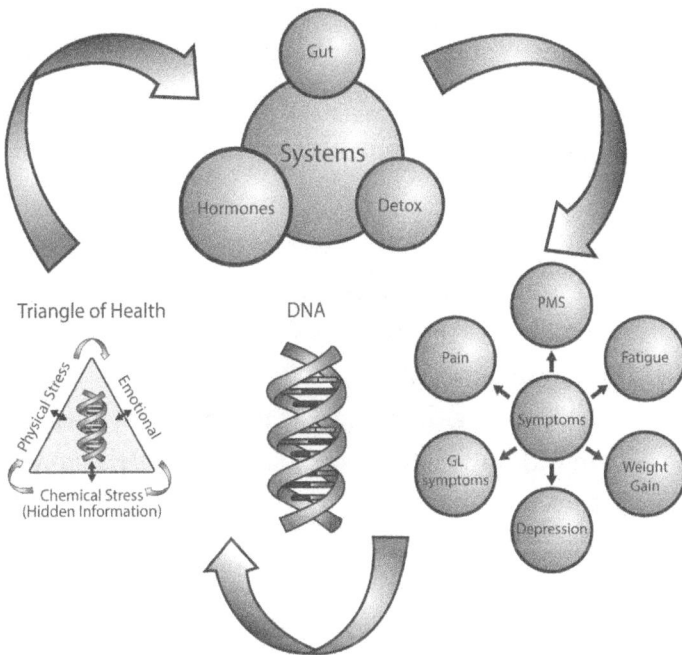

Triangle of Health — Physical Stress — Emotional — Chemical Stress (Hidden Information)

DNA

Systems — Gut — Hormones — Detox

Symptoms — PMS — Pain — Fatigue — GL symptoms — Weight Gain — Depression

Emotional stress includes stress in relationships, finances, family, friends, work, and so on. Or maybe you're just sick and tired of being sick and tired. These are all strong emotional stressors that can keep us from feeling optimal.

Physical stress can be from too little exercise—you're sitting down all day; you're sedentary—or it can be from exercising too much. Maybe you are doing CrossFit or overdoing it as you train for a marathon. Physical stress can also be an unresolved injury (e.g., a back injury or an old knee injury) that's keeping you in pain.

Most of us are familiar with emotional and physical stressors, but there's one more on the triangle, and that is chemical stress—also known as hidden stress because we may not be aware it exists.

Chemical Stressors Can Involve a Variety of Possibilities

These possibilities include the following:

- Nutritional deficiencies needed for healthy thyroid function, like iodine, tyrosine, zinc, selenium, or magnesium
- Blood sugar imbalances
- Food allergies like gluten, dairy, and soy, to name a few
- Gut infections and dysbiosis or SIBO (imbalances in your gut bacteria)
- Malabsorption (taking in enough nutrients but not properly absorbing them)
- Low stomach acid and enzymes
- Insulin resistance and blood sugar imbalances
- Poor sleep and recovery
- Exposure to toxins like alcohol, tobacco, drugs, pesticides, and mold toxins; exogenous hormones in your food; or excessive fluoride from drinking water[31]

The idea in the Triangle of Health is that all the stressors accumulate. If we have chemical stress from consuming gluten and alcohol, this chemical stress from your diet may create excessive inflammation that leaves your joints extra sore. The physical stress from sore joints may keep us from doing things we enjoy, like playing with our kids. Not doing the things you love may cause emotional stress.

You can see how the stressors on the Triangle of Health can literally impact one another: creating inflammation on one side spills into the other side of the triangle, and soon enough, all of these stressors have reached the top of your stress bucket, causing it to overflow (see the image below).

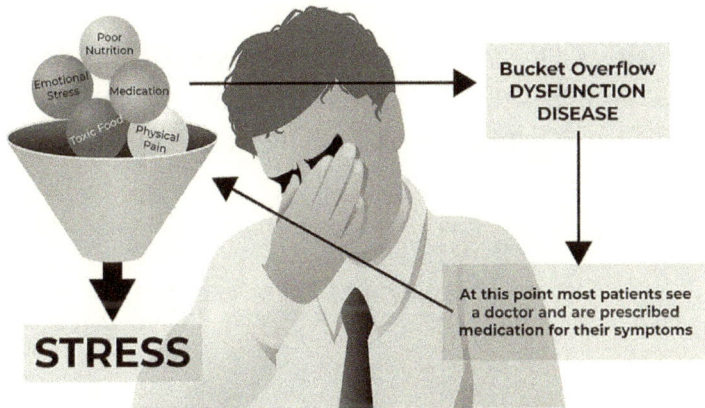

Poor Nutrition

Emotional Stress

Medication

Toxic Food

Physical Pain

**Bucket Overflow
DYSFUNCTION
DISEASE**

At this point most patients see a doctor and are prescribed medication for their symptoms

STRESS

Stressors may be referred to as the *allostatic load*, but I prefer to call this a *stress bucket* because this provides a clear vision of how stress can fill up, overflow, and create symptoms in your life. When the stress bucket overflows, that's when your body systems start to malfunction and create downstream symptoms.

Body Systems

During a review of the body's systems, your practitioner will look for signs of thyroid dysfunction. The systems focused on will include the following:

- Hormonal system (adrenals, thyroid, and male or female hormones)
- Digestive system
- Immune system
- Detoxification system

There's a difference between signs and symptoms. Medical signs are things that can be seen clinically. Symptoms are things you may feel, but they may be harder to verify, like depression or anxiety.

3 BODY SYSTEMS

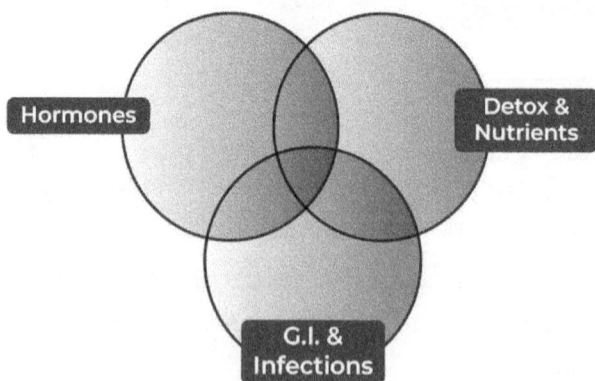

Hormones

Detox & Nutrients

G.I. & Infections

Specific signs may present as the thinning of the outer third of the eyebrow, pale skin, or vertical or horizontal ridges in the fingernails (indicating protein malabsorption). You might be consuming inadequate amounts of protein, have poor digestion due to a gut infection, and have low stomach acid. This can create malabsorption and the inability to break down the protein and utilize it for healthy thyroid and hormonal function. Each system affects the other, and once the body's systems become overwhelmed, we start having symptoms.

Symptoms

There are many symptoms that could result when you have a thyroid disorder, and a good functional medicine practitioner will review these during an exam. In functional medicine, we don't look at symptoms with the goal of prescribing a drug or a supplement to cover them up. We look only at the symptoms to trace them backward, upstream, to the body systems that may not be functioning properly.

Common symptoms of thyroid disorder include:

- Chronic fatigue
- Difficulty losing weight
- Depression
- Muscle or joint aches
- Low libido
- Cold all the time
- Water retention
- Dry skin

- Eczema
- Fibromyalgia
- PMS
- Menopause
- Diffuse hair loss or dry hair
- Cold extremities
- Constipation
- Poor memory
- Poor concentration
- Anxiety
- Weakness
- Shortness of breath
- Palpitations
- Heavy menstrual flow
- Poor motivation

In the Triangle of Health, before a thyroid issue ever comes to light, the first dominos to fall are the individual *stressors*. The second domino is when the body systems become overwhelmed and start to dysfunction. Last but not least, symptoms begin to manifest downstream. This is the general pattern most patients go through: fatigue, cold hands, cold feet, anxiety, depression, and brain fog. These symptoms tend to occur years after the stressors accumulate and affect the body's systems.

The Conventional versus the Functional Approach

The typical conventional medicine approach is to treat each symptom one by one. So if there is depression, for example, you'd get an antidepressant. If there are hormonal symptoms, like PMS, you might get a prescription for birth control. Even natural medicine is guilty of choosing herbs and nutrients to do the same thing, symptom spot treatment, which is much safer than medication. Though this might relieve some symptoms, it doesn't address the root cause or alleviate the problem long term.

In functional medicine, it may be necessary to treat the symptoms temporarily. And that's OK as long as the long-term goal is to eliminate the underlying stress and heal the body's systems and the root cause. The key is to treat and heal holistically, addressing diet, lifestyle, stress management, sleep, blood sugar, adrenals, thyroid, infections, gut bacteria imbalance, toxins, and so on. If we eliminate the stressors and treat the body systems that aren't functioning properly, the symptoms will eventually heal.

Thyroid Lab Testing

I had a patient named Mary come into my office one day. She was complaining of low thyroid symptoms, yet her TSH looked perfect on her thyroid labs, right around 1.5. Her doctor didn't bother ordering her a complete thyroid panel, so the first thing we did was get a complete thyroid panel. Once the results came back, it was clear to see she had elevated TPO antibodies, which meant there was an autoimmune attack occurring and her thyroid was inflamed. She also had T3-free (active thyroid hormone) levels in the bottom 10 percent of the lab reference range at 2.4. This would be within the normal lab range for conventional medicine but outside of the optimal health range that we use in functional medicine. Because we use optimal health ranges instead of disease ranges, we are able to pick up issues sooner.

For thyroid testing, there are optimal or ideal lab ranges (used in functional medicine) as well as standard lab ranges (used in conventional medicine) for the same tests.

Standard lab ranges are created by basically lumping 95 percent of the population together as normal. The remaining 5 percent is considered not normal and is broken into 2.5 percent high and 2.5 percent low.

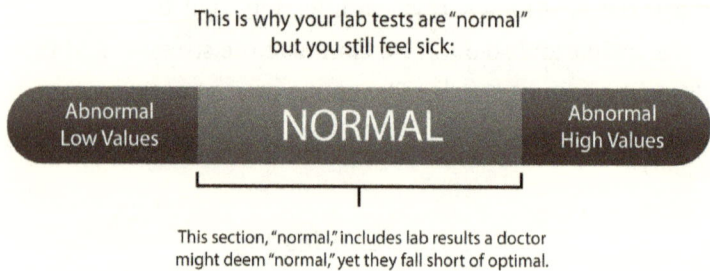

This is why your lab tests are "normal" but you still feel sick:

Abnormal Low Values	NORMAL	Abnormal High Values

This section, "normal," includes lab results a doctor might deem "normal," yet they fall short of optimal.

The problem with the bell curve is that as the general population gets sicker, the so-called normal range must get wider to compensate. If we look at chronic degenerative diseases over the last three or four decades, we see more cancer, more heart disease, more obesity, more diabetes, and so on.

If we know more people are dying of chronic diseases, what does this mean for our lab reference ranges? The wider our so-called normal ranges become, the more people with health challenges (symptoms) are guaranteed to be caught somewhere in the middle. The problem with this is that their doctors will tell them they are fine, it's all in their heads, or they're just getting older. Essentially, people are being told to go home, get sicker, and then years down the road, you may finally test positive with a diagnosed problem. This method wastes too much time and causes too much pain and suffering in the process.

Functional medicine looks at the ideal normal range to get an earlier indicator of potential thyroid dysfunction or imbalance. These ideal ranges are narrower, allowing us to look at someone's thyroid on a spectrum of health rather than simply treating the disease.

This is why your lab tests are "normal" but you still feel sick:

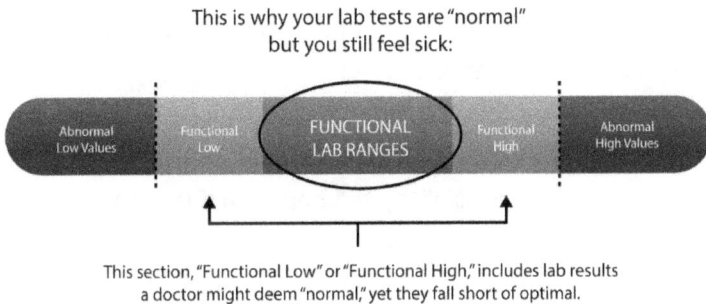

| Abnormal Low Values | Functional Low | FUNCTIONAL LAB RANGES | Functional High | Abnormal High Values |

This section, "Functional Low" or "Functional High," includes lab results a doctor might deem "normal," yet they fall short of optimal.

Imagine a health assessment scale ranging from 1 (representing disease) to 10 (indicating optimal health). Your primary care physician (PCP) is satisfied as long as you're not at 1, the disease state, even if symptoms typically emerge between 5 and 6 on this scale. Despite expressing concerns about not feeling well, if you haven't reached 1, your PCP might still consider you fine. This approach contrasts sharply with that of a functional medicine doctor, who has a different perspective on health. Conventional doctors may view you as normal if no disease is detected, relying on technology and health philosophies that may not be sensitive enough to detect early signs of decline. As a result, you might be advised to return in a year, hoping for answers to explain why you feel the way you feel and a comprehensive treatment plan to fix it.

In functional medicine, we use the ideal range that's more sensitive, and we test more than just the TSH. We also look at T4 total and free, T3 total and free, T3 uptake, reverse T3, thyroid antibodies, thyroglobulin antibodies (TG ab), and thyroid peroxidase antibodies (TPO ab). If we measure all these markers, we get a better window into the thyroid gland's overall function. This also helps us confirm if there is an active autoimmune condition like Hashimoto's when certain antibodies, like TPO ab and TG ab, are present.

We are aware that the thyroid gland's healthy functional tissues will eventually turn sclerotic and lose their ability to produce healthy levels of thyroid hormone if these antibodies attack it repeatedly over time.

I have a reference handout on lab testing, that you are welcome to download. It's located in the resources section at the end of the book.

Thyroid-Stimulating Hormone (TSH)
Standard normal range: 0.5–4.5 mIU/L
Ideal healthy range: 0.5–2.5 mIU/L

TSH is a pituitary hormone that signals the thyroid to make T4. It is a poor measure for estimating the clinical and metabolic severity of primary overt thyroid failure. However, conventional medicine primarily uses it as the only thyroid test. Typically, if TSH drops low (meaning thyroid hormone is high), it's a way of diagnosing hyperthyroidism or even Graves' disease. If TSH levels become elevated (typically meaning T4 and T3 thyroid hormones drop), there could be a deficiency in iodine or an active autoimmune issue, resulting in thyroid swelling or inflammation.

The problem with TSH is that it's a screening test, and it takes many, many years for it to elevate. So a problem can be building for years before testing by conventional medicine discovers it.

If TSH is elevated, we know there's definitely a problem with the thyroid gland. The standard TSH test, however, misses a potential thyroid condition because of how wide the TSH reference has gotten over time. However, if they had looked at the downstream hormones, they could have seen significant imbalances in T4, T3, thyroid antibody levels, and even T3 uptake.

In 2002, a study on thyroid test outcomes from a large sample of individuals representing the US population was published.[32] The research discovered that the typical TSH level (an indicator of thyroid health) is around 1.5 mIU/L. Due to this finding, some organizations have proposed reducing the upper boundary of the normal TSH range. The American Association of Clinical Endocrinology set this limit at 3 mIU/L, while other groups have proposed 2.5 mIU/L. The National Academy of Clinical Biochemistry recommended 4 mIU/L.[33]

Using a narrower TSH range can be super helpful in assessing if you have good thyroid function. When I start to see TSH go to 3 mIU/L or above, I become a little bit suspicious that there may be an underlying thyroid condition starting to develop.

According to survey data from 2007, when TSH goes out of range, TSH levels are correlated with TPO ab positivity.[34] So when your TSH starts to go a little high, you need to test thyroid antibodies to be safe.

Once a patient is on thyroid hormone, you should be very careful relying only on TSH to assess whether thyroid function is optimal. Some studies show TSH levels may not be a great indicator of adequate levels of thyroid hormone systemically in the body, as the receptors in the pituitary are more sensitive to thyroid hormone than the rest of the body is to thyroid hormone.[35] This may cause the TSH levels to be slightly lower than they should be, allowing your T4 and T3 thyroid hormones to get into the upper half of the functional range.

All this means is don't get overly caught up on TSH to assess if you are taking enough thyroid hormone. We don't want to suppress TSH too low on average, like below 0.5 mIU/L; just ensure you get a complete picture of what is happening downstream by including body temperature and how you feel in the overall assessment. It's possible to have a perfect TSH level and thyroid symptoms like fatigue and low body temperature.

Thyroxine (T4) Total
Standard normal range: 4.5–12 μg/dL
Ideal healthy range: 6–10 μg/dL

When we look at hormones individually, we break them into *free* and *protein-bound forms*. A *total* T4 count consists of 98 percent protein-bound hormone, the type of hormone that can't bind to a receptor site, and 2 percent free hormone, which is the part of the hormone that can actually bind to a receptor and create a cellular response in the body.

A protein-bound hormone functions as if you were trying to write with a pen cap on. You can't write—the ink doesn't make contact with the paper, so nothing happens. The pen cap has to be off for that pen to work.

Total T4 is when we look at both free (2 percent) and protein-bound (98 percent), which equals 100 percent of the T4 hormone.

Thyroxine (T4) Free
Standard normal range: 0.8–1.7 ng/dl
Ideal healthy range: 1–1.5 ng/dl

The *free* T4, which represents 2 percent of all T4, provides a positive impact on overall cellular metabolism, including energy, hair, gut function, and mood—all the things that are important for optimal health.

The thyroid then converts 20 percent of that T4 into T3. And then the other 80 percent, as mentioned earlier, gets converted peripherally throughout the body—in the liver, gut, and by healthy adrenal stress hormone levels.

When we test T4 levels, we want to see an ideal total T4 in the range of 6 to 10 µg/dL and a free T4 in the range of 1 to 1.5 µg/dL. Levels outside of these ranges are flags that something is going on with the thyroid.

Free Thyroxine Index (FTI, also referred to as T7)
Standard normal range: 4–11

FTI is an indirect marker calculated based on T3 uptake and total thyroxine levels. FTI, when it's higher, can indicate hyperthyroidism, and a lower FTI can indicate hypothyroidism.

> I don't typically like indirect markers; I prefer to look at the active thyroid hormones.

Triiodothyronine (T3) Total
Standard normal range: 71–180 ng/dL
Ideal healthy range: 100–160 ng/dL

When we look at T3, your active thyroid hormone, we also have to break it into the same *free* and *protein* percentages as T4. The *total* T3 (98 percent protein-bound plus 2 percent free) and free T3 are going to be one of the main tests we look at.

As with free T4, the free T3 levels are always going to be the most important to look at. But it's also good to look at the total T3 just to get a window on how the gland is functioning and producing thyroid hormone.

T3 is going to be the most important level to focus on. One of the major issues that we see is when T4 does not appropriately convert to T3, and there are many reasons why this happens. Factors that can affect conversion include the following:

- Protein deficiency
- Selenium deficiency
- Zinc or magnesium deficiency
- Low iron or ferritin levels
- Low B_{12} levels
- Imbalanced insulin levels or insulin resistance
- Imbalanced cortisol levels
- Increased inflammation

- Gut infections and leaky gut
- Toxins like heavy metals or mycotoxins from mold or pesticides

Triiodothyronine (T3) Free
Standard normal range: 2–4.4 pg/ml
Ideal healthy range: 3–4.2 pg/ml

Free T3 represents about 2 percent of the total T3 production. The free part of the T3 hormone is unbound by the proteins that transport it. This small amount of unbound hormone is the portion of T3 that the body actually uses and has access to. When free T3 is at proper levels, this enhances energy, mood, hair, skin, and so many other things that make us feel good and keep our bodies at optimal function.

When we test T3 levels, we want to see an ideal total T3 in the range of 100 to 160 ng/dL, and an ideal free T3 in the range of 3 to 4 pg/ml. Levels outside of these ranges are a red flag that something is going on with the thyroid.

When we see T3-free levels below 3, a natural thyroid glandular or thyroid medication like Armour, NP Thyroid, WP Thyroid, or Nature Thyroid may be necessary. Before recommending a thyroid glandular, it's important to make sure all of the above nutrients and critical barriers to healing are supported. We also want to see if the patient has any low thyroid symptoms before we jump in to provide additional support. There are other factors that need to be taken into account, like TSH levels, adrenal levels, and thyroid antibody levels.

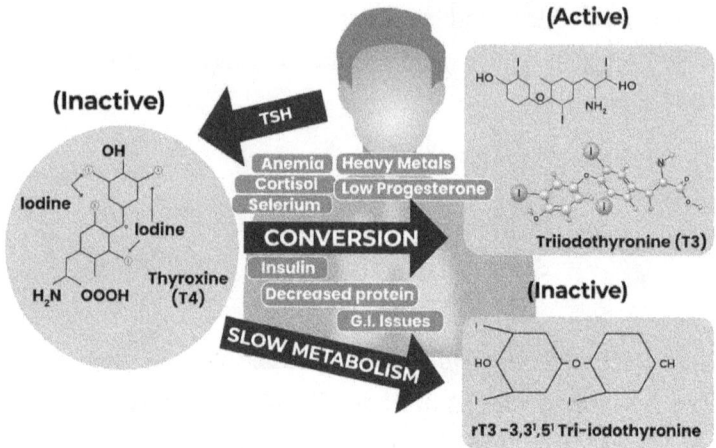

T3 Uptake

Standard normal range: 24–39 percent
Ideal healthy range: 27–37 percent

T3 uptake looks at how the body is able to utilize thyroid hormone indirectly by measuring the binding capacity of thyroid-binding globulin (more on this later).

In other words, when thyroid-binding protein drops, T3 free increases, thus causing a higher T3 uptake. Factors that increase T3 uptake are elevated androgens, like in PCOS (polycystic ovary syndrome), and corticosteroids, including prednisone.

When thyroid-binding protein increases, T3 free drops, thus causing a lower T3 uptake. Factors that decrease T3 uptake include birth control, other hormone-based contraceptives, or exogenous hormones in the environment (food, water, etc.).

Reverse T3

Standard normal range: 9–24.1 ng/dl
Ideal healthy range: 14.9–22 ng/dl

Reverse T3 is equivalent to metabolic blanks in your thyroid gun, so to speak. Reverse T3 binds to the thyroid receptor site just like T3 free, without the same metabolic response. This is just like putting a blank in a real gun; when you pull the trigger, there is a loud noise but no bullet. Elevated cortisol levels due to adrenal stress can contribute to high reverse T3 levels.

Lower reverse T3 levels are a sign of stress, a slower metabolism, and potentially lower iodine levels. The more stress we have, the more T4 converts to reverse T3 instead of healthy active T3. Finding reverse T3 outside of the ideal normal range would alert the functional medicine practitioner that there is stress that needs to be addressed.

Thyroid Peroxidase Antibody (TPO ab)

Standard normal range: 0–15 IU/ml
Ideal healthy range: 0–15 IU/ml

Like TG ab, the presence of TPO ab above the normal range should raise suspicion of autoimmunity or Hashimoto's. The immune system also calls on this antibody to fight the thyroid when it mistakenly sees it as an invader, and it needs to be addressed before the body can do too much damage to itself. Patients with TPO ab, as I mentioned previously, can also have elevated TG ab, so it's good to run both. Some may even switch back and forth between the two antibodies.

Thyroglobulin Antibody
(TG ab or Antithyroglobulin)
Standard normal range: 0–0.9 IU/ml
Ideal healthy range: 0–0.9 IU/ml

The presence of the TG ab above the normal range should raise suspicion of autoimmunity or Hashimoto's. The immune system calls on this antibody to fight the thyroid when it mistakenly sees it as an invader, and it needs to be addressed before the body can do too much damage to itself. Patients with TG ab can also have TPO ab. Some may even switch back and forth.

Thyroid-Binding Globulin (TBG)
Standard normal range: 13–39 mcg/dL
Ideal healthy range: 18–27 mcg/dL

TBG is a binding protein that binds to thyroid hormone to help transport it throughout the body. Certain situations can increase thyroid-binding globulin levels, like pregnancy, birth control, or other hormone contraceptives. If you are on additional hormones, adding TBG to your thyroid panel would be a good idea. As you increase TBG, you will typically see the T3 free and T4 free levels drop correspondingly.

TBG can drop with exposure to corticosteroids and prednisone. High levels of androgens or testosterone, like those seen in PCOS (polycystic ovary syndrome), can lower TBG as well. Low levels of protein, liver stress, and kidney stress can also decrease TBG.

Thyroglobulin (TG is not to be confused with TBG)
Standard normal range: 1–10 ng/mL
Suggestive of malignancy: above 10 ng/mL

TG is the form that thyroid hormone takes when it is stored in the thyroid tissue or follicle. The TG test is typically ordered to rule out thyroid cancer and thyroid nodules. TG may also be ordered to monitor the thyroid post-cancer or if your thyroid has been ablated with radioactive iodine treatment.

Thyroid Temperature Testing

Thyroid temperature is important because heat is one of the by-products of metabolism. We can use basal body temperature as an indirect measure of how someone's thyroid gland is functioning.

You can measure your thyroid temperature using a good-quality fertility digital thermometer. Place the thermometer either in your armpit or in your mouth. A healthy thyroid temperature range, if you're using the axillary or armpit area, is 97.8 to 98.2 degrees. If you're measuring by mouth, it is 98.2 to 98.6 degrees.

Check the temperature first thing in the morning each day to see if it is consistently in that healthy range. Do this before you get out of bed and start moving around. If your temperature is dropping or fluctuating by more than 0.3 degrees each day, you may have some type of adrenal stress (high or low cortisol rhythm imbalance), even if your temperature is in the normal range.

If the temperature runs chronically low without fluctuations (e.g., 97.2 or 96.8), that's a sign of low thyroid function. This type of testing is not an exact science but can provide a noninvasive, inexpensive way to assess your thyroid function. You always want to follow up with thyroid blood testing to be certain.

For a woman, thyroid temperature testing can be done on days two to six of her cycle. Since her temperature will drop before ovulation and rise again when she enters the luteal phase (the second half of her cycle), measuring her temperature early on will help get an accurate reading without the interference of other hormones that can increase her metabolism, like progesterone. Looking at those first five days after her period can be really helpful in getting a good sense of what her temperature is without other hormones influencing it.

I have handouts on the procedure for temperature testing, "Basal Temperature Instructions," that you are welcome to download. These handouts are located in the resources section at the end of the chapter and the book.

Other Tests for the Thyroid

Other tests your functional medicine practitioner might perform include palpating the thyroid, which simply means manually feeling or pressing externally to check for asymmetry, nodules, or bumps. Up to 10 percent of thyroid autoimmunity blood testing can come back with a false negative, meaning the test is showing negative but the person really is positive for Hashimoto's.[36] When the practitioner feels they may be getting a false negative, the patient can be sent for an ultrasound to see if anything comes up there. If the exam, lab work, and ultrasound are all coming back clean, it's unlikely there is an autoimmune condition present. I typically assume there is an autoimmune issue in the beginning when dealing with patients with thyroid symptoms.

The last way to confirm Hashimoto's is through a needle biopsy. I do not typically recommend this unless we are trying to rule out some type of thyroid cancer.

You can order your own thyroid test with all of the markers mentioned above by visiting the site in the resources section or at the end of the chapter.

When Is the Best Time to Test Your Thyroid?

Testing thyroid hormone in the morning is the best time, as your metabolism is increased as you start your day. It's good to have a consistent time as your metabolism may fluctuate later in the day, so be consistent with your testing time.

When conducting a thyroid test, I aim to gauge a patient's optimal thyroid hormone levels accurately. It's fine to eat breakfast thirty to sixty minutes after taking your thyroid medication. Breakfast can stimulate metabolism, leading to more precise thyroid test results that reflect a patient's everyday routine, assuming they normally eat breakfast (which is advised). Contrary to the common recommendation from many doctors to avoid food before thyroid testing—which might artificially reduce thyroid hormone levels and increase TSH—I believe eating is preferable, unless you usually practice intermittent fasting in the mornings. In my clinical experience, consuming breakfast provides a better indication of daily hormone levels.

It's also important to avoid acid reflux medications and minerals like iron and calcium, as they can impact thyroid hormone absorption. Avoid biotin as well as it can elevate T4 and T3, and lower TSH falsely.

Many doctors recommend taking thyroid glandular or natural desiccated thyroid (NDT) supplements after a thyroid function test. This advice is particularly applicable if you are on a T4-only medication regimen. T4, the main hormone prescribed by most traditional medical professionals, has a half-life of four to six days, meaning its levels remain relatively stable over time. In contrast, T3, which is present in Armour Thyroid and other NDT supplements, has a much shorter half-life—ranging from six to twenty-four hours. This can lead to significant fluctuations in hormone levels, with some patients metabolizing most of their T3 by noon (as shown in the graph below). I've observed patients who, when tested in the morning on an empty stomach, have T3 levels comparable to those before they even began regular thyroid support. This suggests that their bodies have already metabolized all the T3, rendering morning tests before taking NDT an inaccurate reflection of their actual thyroid hormone levels throughout the day, typically showing lower than actual levels.

My goal is to see T3-free levels at or above 3.0 pg/ml, at a minimum of the top 50 percent of the reference range, ideally reaching into the top 25 percent of the reference range and even a little higher as you may be there for only a short period of time before your hormone levels start to naturally come down. This is OK as long as the TSH looks good, it's not below 0.5, and there are no hyperthyroid symptoms like excessive sweating, irritability, insomnia, heart palpitations, or anxiety. Doctors need to ensure they aren't just looking at the labs; how the patient feels is just as important. Looking at basal body temperatures can also be another good indicator to add to the mix when assessing optimal thyroid dosage.

If I see patients testing on the higher side of T3 free (mid to upper 4.0 pg/ml) with adequate TSH (0.5 to 2.5 mIU/L), I will typically have those patients wait until after a thyroid test to take their first morning thyroid dose. This is because these patients may be slower metabolizers of T3 and will still have some thyroid in their system from the previous afternoon's dose, giving a false high reading.

Philosophically, my goal is to get a window or snapshot of where a patient's T3-free levels are on average throughout the day. Most patients on a dose above 0.5 grains or higher report feeling better taking their thyroid hormone two times throughout the day, providing better all-day coverage. In addition, this prevents a drop in the last half of the day, which may help improve energy and mood.

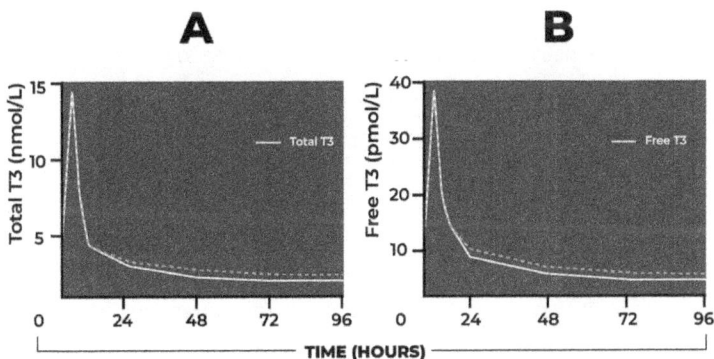

Thyroid Health and Healing

We'll explore thyroid health and healing options in depth when we delve into later chapters. Briefly, we want to do the following to assure thyroid health and healing:

- Make sure your diet is anti-inflammatory and nutrient dense
- Get your gut functioning correctly
- Eliminate infections
- Properly manage your stress
- Address adrenal function
- Eliminate or limit gluten consumption
- Limit toxins to de-stress your liver and detoxification system
- Apply natural, functional medicine treatments
- Get to the root cause of your thyroid issue

KEY POINTS

1. The main function of the thyroid gland is to serve as the center of metabolism, which has an impact on every cell in the body. It can impact body temperature, energy, mood, bowel regularity, weight, hair, and skin, to name a few.

2. Twenty percent of thyroid hormone conversion (T4 to T3) happens in the thyroid. The other 80 percent

happens in the liver and in the gut, depending on stress levels.

3. Iodine, tyrosine, and selenium are the main elements for thyroid hormone production. However, there is a fine balance between too much and too little.

4. Most thyroid conditions are the result of a root cause that resides somewhere else in the body. Finding the root cause is the key to supporting optimal thyroid function.

5. Standard lab ranges, typically used by conventional medicine, can be too wide and can delay the diagnosis of a thyroid condition by years. It is best to look at ideal lab ranges used in functional medicine and address thyroid issues before they become out of control.

Resources

Access to Dr. J (www.justinhealth.com/free-consult) Here you can find virtual options to work with me if you want to dive in as a patient and get to the root of your thyroid and other health challenges.

Thyroid Reboot Foundations Bundle (www.justinhealth.com/foundations) Here are several recommended thyroid-supporting supplements mentioned in the book in easy-to-access bundles.

Access to the Thyroid Course (www.justinhealth.com/thyroid-course) Here you can find my course, which is an in-depth video version of this course in a live-lecture format. There are live Q & As to enhance your experience of the book.

Basal Temperature Instructions (www.justinhealth.com/temperature-test) This is an easy handout to chart your basal body temperature and assess your metabolism.

Blood Test Review (www.justinhealth.com/blood-test-road-map) This is an Excel sheet that contains the reference range for thyroid labs as well as other blood tests I use.

Complete Thyroid Test (www.justinhealth.com/complete-thyroid-test) This is a comprehensive thyroid panel, including TSH, T4 free, T4 total, T3 free, T3 total, TPO ab, TG ab, and RT3.

Abridged Thyroid Test (www.justinhealth.com/abridged-thyroid-test) This is an abridged thyroid panel including TSH, T4 free, T3 free, TPO ab, and TG ab.

Thyroid Laser (www.justinhealth.com/thyroid-laser) Here you will be able to get information on purchasing or renting a therapeutic grade laser to help with thyroid inflammation and stimulate thyroid tissue healing.

Notes

1   Theodore C. Friedman and David R. Cool, "Prohormones," *Encyclopedia of Endocrine Diseases* (2004): 91–98, https://doi.org/10.1016/B0-12-475570-4/01074-X.

2   Wilmar M. Wiersinga et al., ""2012 ETA Guidelines: The Use of L-T4 + L-T3 in the Treatment of Hypothyroidism,"" *European Thyroid Journal* 1, no. 2 (2012): 55–71, https://doi.org/10.1159/000339444.

3   M. T. Hays, "Thyroid Hormone and the Gut," *Endocrine Research* 14, no. 2–3 (1988): 203–224, https://doi.org/10.3109/07435808809032986.
4   Hays.
5   Robin P. Peeters and Theo J. Visser, "Metabolism of Thyroid Hormone," in *Endotext*, K. R. Feingold et al., eds. (South Dartmouth, MA: MDText.com, 2000), https://www.ncbi.nlm.nih.gov/books/NBK285545.
6   David V. Becker et al., ""Iodine Supplementation for Pregnancy and Lactation — United States and Canada: Recommendations of the American Thyroid Association,"" *Thyroid* 16, no. 10 (2006): 949–51, https://doi.org/10.1089/thy.2006.16.949.
7   American Thyroid Association. ""Hypothyroidism: First-Degree Family Members of Patients with Hypothyroidism Due to Hashimoto's Thyroiditis Have an Increased Risk of Developing Hypothyroidism," *Clinical Thyroidology for the Public* 10, no. 9 (September 2017): 8–9, https://www.thyroid.org/patient-thyroid-information/ct-for-patients/september-2017/vol-10-issue-9-p-8-9.
8   Xiaoming Lou et al., "The Effect of Iodine Status on the Risk of Thyroid Nodules: A Cross-Sectional Study in Zhejiang, China," *International Journal of Endocrinology* 2020 (August 18, 2020): 3760375, https://doi.org/10.1155/2020/3760375.
9   N. Konno et al., "Association between Dietary Iodine Intake and Prevalence of Subclinical Hypothyroidism in the Coastal Regions of Japan," *Journal of Clinical Endocrinology & Metabolism* 78, no. 2 (February 1994): 393–97, https://doi.org/10.1210/jcem.78.2.8106628.
10 Hoji Suzuki et al., "Endemic Coast Goitre in Hokkaido, Japan," *Acta Endocrinologica* 50, no. 2 (October 1965): 161–76, https://doi.org/10.1530/acta.0.0500161.
11 Nobuyuki Amino, "Autoimmunity and Hypothyroidism," *Baillière's Clinical Endocrinology and Metabolism* 2, no. 3 (August 1988): 591–617, https://doi.org/10.1016/S0950-351X(88)80055-7.
12 B. Corvilain et al., "Selenium and the Thyroid: How the Relationship Was Established," *American Journal of Clinical Nutrition* 57, no. 2 (February 1993): 244S–48S, https://doi.org/10.1093/ajcn/57.2.244S.
13 E. B. Astwood, Carl E. Cassidy, and G. D. Aurbach, "Treatment of Goiter and Thyroid Nodules with Thyroid," *Journal of the American Medical Association* 174, no. 5 (1960): 459–64, https://doi.org/10.1001/jama.1960.03030050001001.

14 Iyshwarya Bhaskar Kalarani and Ramakrishnan Veerabathiran, "Impact of Iodine Intake on the Pathogenesis of Autoimmune Thyroid Disease in Children and Adults," *Annals of Pediatric Endocrinology & Metabolism* 27, no. 4 (2022): 256–64, https://doi.org/10.6065/apem.2244186.093; and Jiameng Liu et al., "Excessive Iodine Promotes Pyroptosis of Thyroid Follicular Epithelial Cells in Hashimoto's Thyroiditis through the ROS-Nf-kB-NLRP3 Pathway," *Frontiers in Endocrinology* 10 (2019), https://doi.org/10.3389/fendo.2019.00778.

15 Marta Rydzewska et al., "Role of the T and B Lymphocytes in Pathogenesis of Autoimmune Thyroid Diseases," *Thyroid Research* 11 (2018): 2, https://doi.org/10.1186/s13044-018-0046-9.

16 Nikoo Hossein-Khannazer et al., ""Low-Level Laser Therapy in the Treatment of Autoimmune Thyroiditis," *Journal of Lasers in Medical Sciences* 13, no. 10 (2022): e34, https://doi.org/10.34172%2Fjlms.2022.34.

17 Theodore T. Zava and David T. Zava, "Assessment of Japanese Iodine Intake Based on Seaweed Consumption in Japan: A Literature-Based Analysis," *Thyroid Research* 4 (2011): 14, https://doi.org/10.1186/1756-6614-4-14.

18 Dr. David Brownstein, "Busting the Iodine Myths – by Dr. David Brownstein," *Power2Practice* (blog), January 10, 2017, https://www.power2practice.com/article/busting-the-iodine-myths/; and Datis Kharrazian, ""Iodine and Hashimoto's,"" Kharrazian Resource Center, November 28, 2012, https://drknews.com/iodine-and-hashimotos.

19 Patrizio Caturegli et al., "Hashimoto's Thyroiditis: Celebrating the Centennial through the Lens of the Johns Hopkins Hospital Surgical Pathology Records," *Thyroid* 23, no. 2 (2013), https://doi.org/10.1089/thy.2012.0554.

20 Caturegli et al.

21 Salvatore Benvenga and Fabrizio Guarneri, "Molecular Mimicry and Autoimmune Thyroid Disease," *Reviews in Endocrine and Metabolic Disorders* 17 (2016): 485–98, https://doi.org/10.1007/s11154-016-9363-2.

22 Maarten P. Rozing et al., "Serum Triiodothyronine Levels and Inflammatory Cytokine Production Capacity," *AGE* 34 (2012): 195–201, https://doi.org/10.1007/s11357-011-9220-x.

23 Piotr Kocełak et al., "Anti-Thyroid Antibodies in the Relation to TSH Levels and Family History of Thyroid Diseases in Young Caucasian Women," *Frontiers in Endocrinology* 13 (December 19, 2022), https://doi.org/10.3389/fendo.2022.1081157.

24 Kocełak et al.

25 Hannah Nieto and Kristien Boelaert, ""Women In Cancer Thematic Review: Thyroid-Stimulating Hormone in Thyroid Cancer: Does It Matter?,"" *Endocrine-Related Cancer* 23, no. 11 (November 2016): T109–21, https://doi.org/10.1530/ERC-16-0328.

26 Xiaojie Hu et al., "Cancer Risk in Hashimoto's Thyroiditis: A Systematic Review and Meta-Analysis," *Frontiers in Endocrinology* 13 (July 12, 2022), https://doi.org/10.3389/fendo.2022.937871.

27 Alessandro Antonelli et al., "Graves' Disease: Epidemiology, Genetic and Environmental Risk Factors and Viruses," *Best Practice & Research Clinical Endocrinology & Metabolism* 34, no. 1 (January 2020): 101387, https://doi.org/10.1016/j.beem.2020.101387.

28 Indu Khurana, Arushi Khurana, and Narayan Gurukripa Kowlgi, *Textbook of Medical Physiology*, 3rd ed., e-book (New Delhi: Reed Elsevier India, 2020).

29 George J. Kahaly et al., "2018 European Thyroid Association Guideline for the Management of Graves' Hyperthyroidism," *European Thyroid Journal* 7, no. 4 (July 25, 2018): 167–86, https://doi.org/10.1159/000490384.

30 Suzuki et al., "'Endemic Coast Goitre' in Hokkaido, Japan."

31 Taiji Liisa Somppi, "Non-Thyroidal Illness Syndrome in Patients Exposed to Indoor Air Dampness Microbiota Treated Successfully with Triiodothyronine," *Frontiers in Immunology* 8 (2017), https://doi.org/10.3389/fimmu.2017.00919.

32 Joseph G. Hollowell et al., "Serum TSH, T4, and Thyroid Antibodies in the United States Population (1988 to 1994): National Health and Nutrition Examination Survey (NHANES III)," *Journal of Clinical Endocrinology & Metabolism* 87, no. 2 (February 1, 2002): 489–99, https://doi.org/10.1210/jcem.87.2.8182.

33 James D. Faix and Linda M. Thienpont, "Thyroid-Stimulating Hormone," Association for Diagnostics & Laboratory Medicine, May 1, 2013, https://www.myadlm.org/cln/articles/2013/may/tsh-harmonization.

34 C. A. Spencer et al., "National Health and Nutrition Examination
Survey III Thyroid-Stimulating Hormone (TSH)-Thyroperoxidase
Antibody Relationships Demonstrate that TSH Upper Limit
Reference Limits May Be Skewed by Occult Thyroid Dysfunction,"
Journal of Clinical Endocrinology & Metabolism 92, no. 11
(November 2007): 4236–40, https://doi.org/10.1210/jc.2007-0287.

35 W. D. Fraser et al., "Are Biochemical Tests of Thyroid Function
of Any Value in Monitoring Patients Receiving Thyroxine
Replacement?," *British Medical Journal (Clinical Research
Edition)* 293 (September 27, 1986): 808, https://doi.org/10.1136/
bmj.293.6550.808.

36 James R. Baker et al., "Seronegative Hashimoto Thyroiditis with
Thyroid Autoantibody Production Localized to the Thyroid,"
Annals of Internal Medicine 108, no. 1 (January 1, 1988): 26–30,
https://doi.org/10.7326/0003-4819-108-1-26.

2

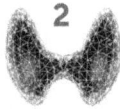

Thyroid-Supporting Diet and Lifestyle

DIET IS AN IMPORTANT FOUNDATIONAL COMPO-
nent when managing thyroid imbalances. Every bite
of food you take puts your body into either an anti-inflammatory state or a pro-inflammatory state. The foods recommended on my meal map are high in quality fats, proteins,
and the right carbohydrates that help you rebuild and heal your
body and lower your inflammation.

Food can also drive you into a pro-inflammatory state. This
occurs when you are consuming more grains, flours, processed
omega-6 fatty acids in refined vegetable oil, and trans fats.
These foods make it extremely hard for you to heal and put you
on an accelerated aging path. When your body makes more
prostaglandin E2 and overproduces interleukins, cytokines,

cortisol, and adrenaline, it becomes harder for you to jump off this fast track to disease.

The thyroid is important for metabolism and generating energy. We need a healthy thyroid diet to metabolize cholesterol, which gets converted into your hormone-building blocks—pregnenolone. Low thyroid levels can cause elevations in cholesterol, which can affect other hormone pathways downstream like estrogen, progesterone, cortisol, and testosterone imbalances.

In addition to diet in this chapter, a good functional medicine practitioner will also look at activity levels and lifestyle (sleep patterns, stress management, hydration, and rest, to name a few), which are also key factors to healing and maintaining a healthy thyroid.

Three Important Criteria for a Thyroid Reboot Diet

When we are dealing with thyroid issues, the following three major characteristics make up the foundation of the thyroid reboot diet:

- **Nutrient density**: A nutrient-dense diet includes foods rich in vitamins, minerals, and antioxidants and which support your body's ability to heal and to run its metabolic pathways optimally.

- **Anti-inflammatory**: An anti-inflammatory diet promotes healing and extinguishes the metabolic fires from the stress of your daily life. It can also help balance the immune system and decrease autoimmune flares.

- **Low in toxins:** A diet low in toxins (e.g., avoiding alcohol, drugs, chlorine, pesticides, fluoride, heavy metals, mycotoxins, etc.) helps relieve stress on your hormonal and detoxification systems. Eating organic vegetables, fruits, starches, fats, and animal proteins will help this.

These three major criteria should form the foundation of your diet. From there, we can manage blood sugar and tweak macronutrients such as proteins, fats, and carbohydrates as needed.

The Blood-Sugar Connection

Blood sugar levels can fluctuate from high to low when certain types of foods are eaten. Typically, these blood sugar swings are caused when excessive amounts of carbohydrates (refined sugars, starch, and grains) are consumed. To make things easier to understand, I will be using the word *sugar* interchangeably with *glucose* and *fructose*.

There weren't the same levels of access to refined carbohydrates for your ancestors just over a hundred years ago. These foods are widely available today in our Standard American Diet (SAD). Our ancestors' diets were typically made up of healthy proteins, fats from animal products (organic and pasture-fed), healthy non-starchy vegetables, and sparing amounts of starchy vegetables, tubers, and fruit. Our diets today are backward from our ancestors' way of life.

Take a look at the consumption of sugar over the last two hundred years. Only a few pounds per year for the average person in the early-to-mid 1800s is now up to over a hundred pounds per year for the average person. And for every healthy person keeping their sugar consumption low, there is a very unhealthy person consuming over two hundred pounds per year.[1] Just crazy!

US Sugar Consumption, 1822–2005

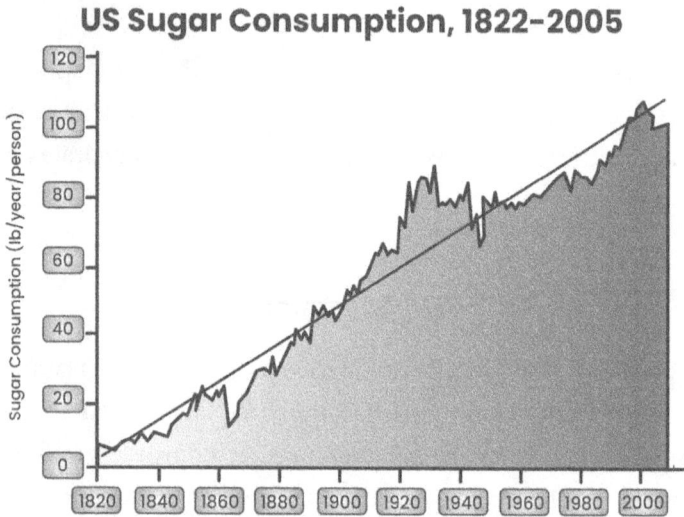

Processed foods like sugar and honey were rare and expensive, making them less accessible to the average person. Now this is not the case. Most governments in the world provide subsidies for these refined, calorie-dense carbohydrates, making them even more affordable and accessible. This easy-to-access, cheap, processed food has only fueled more disease while putting more stress on your thyroid, pancreas, and adrenal glands. These glands play a major role in supporting blood sugar balance.

To keep blood sugar levels stable, sugar should come primarily in the form of non-starchy vegetables, such as broccoli, brussels sprouts, asparagus, cauliflower, and sauerkraut, and low-sugar fruits, such as berries, grapefruit, lemons, limes, and green apples.

If you are coming into this thyroid reboot already overweight, there is a really good chance there is insulin resistance and a metabolic syndrome making your body's receptor sites numb to insulin. If you are numb to insulin, it means you are consuming too much carbohydrate or processed sugar, causing your pancreas to oversecrete insulin, which is a storage hormone. The more insulin your pancreas produces, the more your cells become numb to it. The more numb or resistant to insulin your cells become, the less efficient your body becomes at burning sugar properly. Instead, it gets very good at storing excess glucose, fructose, and carbohydrates as fat, which further slows down your metabolism.

Vegetables, for most people, should be the foundation of the carbohydrate portion of their diet because they are lower in sugar and yet are still very nutrient dense. The blood-sugar connection to a healthy thyroid is vital. We need healthy insulin and blood sugar levels to convert your thyroid hormone from T4, the inactive hormone, to T3, the active hormone. If blood sugar is too high, resulting in too much insulin secretion from the pancreas, that's going to keep the body from activating and converting your thyroid hormone.

Reactive Hypoglycemia

When your blood sugar (also called glucose) goes up and down after eating a meal with excess carbohydrates and refined sugar, this is called *reactive hypoglycemia*. The overreaction of the pancreas to the excess glucose now in your bloodstream makes it "reactive" hypoglycemia. Standard hypoglycemia may be just as bad for you but is primarily due to skipping meals and not eating enough food. Eating the right foods every four to five hours is important (at least initially) because it helps take the stress off your pancreas and adrenal glands by balancing out the highs and lows of your blood sugar swings.

When you eat that extra sugar, your body brings the sugar into your bloodstream really fast. This makes your blood sugar spike, and then your body tells your pancreas to spit out a whole bunch of insulin. This insulin surge drops blood sugar, which then stimulates your adrenal gland to make more cortisol and adrenaline to help pick up your low blood sugar levels. This is the reason why, after a blood sugar crash, you may notice you suddenly feel fatigued, dizzy, irritable, and anxious.

Here's an analogy I give my patients when I talk about blood sugar: Reactive hypoglycemia is like starting and keeping a fire lit with paper and twigs. The fire lights up extremely fast, but within a few minutes, it's out. You find yourself constantly having to feed the fire when you are using this type of fuel source. The twigs and paper are equivalent to the excess refined carbs or sugar in this analogy.

When you use a healthier fuel source for the fire, like a log, the fire burns longer and hotter for hours. Eventually, you will have to add another log to the fire to keep it going, just like having a second meal. The logs on the fire in this analogy are equivalent to healthy proteins and fats, which should make up most of the calories you consume.

It is particularly important to avoid this blood sugar roller coaster if you have thyroid issues. Eating proteins, fats, and the right carbohydrates is the perfect step to moving out of this vicious blood sugar cycle. I have seen many patients stuck in this blood sugar roller coaster cycle for years.

HIGH CARB MEAL & EFFECT ON THYROID FUNCTION

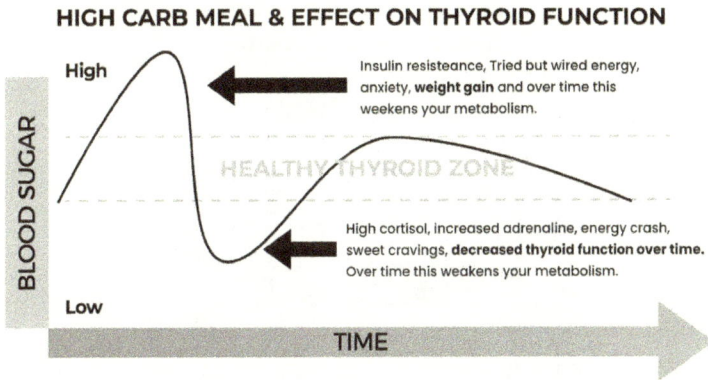

Insulin resisteance, Tried but wired energy, anxiety, **weight gain** and over time this weekens your metabolism.

HEALTHY THYROID ZONE

High cortisol, increased adrenaline, energy crash, sweet cravings, **decreased thyroid function over time.** Over time this weakens your metabolism.

The Proteins, Fats, and Carbs Connection

The graphic is not an exact recommendation but gives good general macronutrient percentages. The range shows about 50 percent fat, 30 percent protein, and 20 percent carbs, give or take ten to twenty in either direction depending on your metabolic type, carb tolerance, and activity levels.

This could put you on a lower-carb, keto paleo template where carbs are at 10 percent, fats at 70 percent, and protein at 20 percent. Or a zone paleo template where carbs may go as high as 40 percent, protein at 30 percent, and fats at 30 percent. This template may be good for those who are trying to gain weight or who are very metabolically active. Proteins, fats, and carbs can be adjusted like a lever and tweaked to meet your exact metabolic needs. I have a general rule with most patients: always start on the lower carb side of the macros, stabilize first, optimize, and adjust carbs upward based on energy, how active you are, and weight loss goals.

General Macronutrient Recommendation

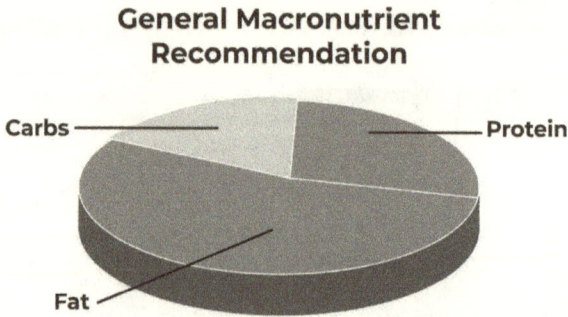

Consuming a healthy balance of macronutrients—proteins, fats, and carbohydrates—is important. Let's say you're eating healthy proteins—beef, chicken, fish, turkey, salmon, and so on. Let's say you're also eating healthy fats—coconut oil, avocado, ghee, or grass-fed butter. But then you go off the deep end with your carbohydrates and eat a lot of grains, high-sugar tropical fruits, or refined-sugar snacks. This will throw off the balance of macronutrients and cause a problem. We need to make sure we have the carbohydrates in check.

Protein Recommendations

I recommend eating one serving size of protein every four or five hours, depending on how active you are; one serving size should measure anywhere between a palm and a fist size or even a full hand (three to eight ounces). Typically, bigger people have bigger hands, so this is a good measurement. The best proteins are typically high-quality animal proteins, and I usually recommend choosing a protein that is full of fat, as long as you're getting it from organic, pasture-fed sources. Toxins tend to concentrate in the fat portion of meats. Choosing proteins from the following types of meat sources gives us the best chance at having less toxicity:

- Beef should be organic, grass-fed meat.
- Fish should be wild, such as Alaska sockeye salmon; skipjack tuna is also good.
- Chicken should be pasture-raised chicken.

The problem with getting your proteins from plant products is that they have to be combined with other carbohydrates to make a complete protein, and plant proteins usually come with a lot of carbohydrates, the exceptions being soy and plant protein powders. Soy has its own whole host of issues due to its estrogenic content and trypsin inhibitors that make digestion more difficult.

For instance, rice and beans need to be combined together to make a complete protein source. The problem with this combination is the amount of carbohydrates. What you get in one cup of rice and beans is about 54 g of carbohydrates per 12 g of protein. You're essentially getting four times as many carbohydrates as protein. So if you're someone who needs 30 to 40 g of protein per meal, you'll be getting an awful lot of carbohydrates. For some people, that may be too many and can drive insulin resistance.

Fat Recommendations

Fat is essential for good health. Fats tell your body you are full and also provide building blocks for hair, skin, and nails. Our cell membranes have a lipid or fat bilayer, which leads to healthy tissues, which leads to a healthy body. Your cells need healthy fats to be healthy.

I recommend three to six ounces of full fat two to three times per day. Animal meats tend to be a great source, so if you're already getting proteins from animal sources, you're also likely getting healthy fats. It's pretty hard to go low-fat with animal proteins unless you choose boneless, skinless chicken breast (I always recommend that if you're doing the chicken breast, keep the skin on and switch to chicken thighs if possible).

If your main source of protein isn't animal meat, you will need to add additional fat to your meals, like avocado. If you use a plant-based protein powder like pea protein, for example, add some unsweetened coconut milk or a scoop of coconut or MCT oil to your protein shake. This will add that extra bit of fat you need to help stabilize your blood sugar and make the meal more balanced. Nuts and seeds will also be an important staple if you can tolerate them. I always recommend eating healthy animal products when they are available due to their increased nutritional density and rich fatty-acid profile.

Carbohydrate Recommendations

Your body can hold roughly 300 to 350 g (grams) of carbohydrates in your muscles, depending on how big they are. When your carbohydrate levels are topped off in your muscles (glycogen), the next place carbohydrates are stored is in your liver.

Your liver can hold only about 60 to 80 g and can become saturated much quicker. Any remaining carbohydrates are converted into fat. Your body is very efficient at turning carbohydrates into fat and will do so if there are too many carbohydrates in your diet.

Do you know how many teaspoons of glucose are typically present in your bloodstream? With about 6 liters of blood in an average person, a glucose level of 100 mg/dL translates to approximately one teaspoon of sugar in your bloodstream. When you drink a 12-ounce Coke, for example, you're ingesting 10 teaspoons of sugar. So where does all that excess sugar, beyond the single teaspoon, go? Your body either converts this glucose into glycogen to store in the muscles and liver, burns it off during exercise, or converts it to fat.

Daily Carbohydrate Recommendations

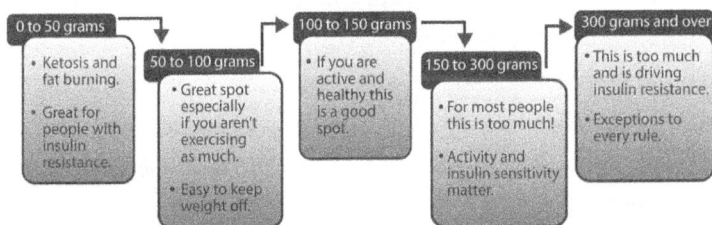

0 to 50 grams
- Ketosis and fat burning.
- Great for people with insulin resistance.

50 to 100 grams
- Great spot especially if you aren't exercising as much.
- Easy to keep weight off.

100 to 150 grams
- If you are active and healthy this is a good spot.

150 to 300 grams
- For most people this is too much!
- Activity and insulin sensitivity matter.

300 grams and over
- This is too much and is driving insulin resistance.
- Exceptions to every rule.

Blood glucose levels are tightly regulated in our bodies. If the concentration drops to half a teaspoon, you could become hypoglycemic, risking a coma. Conversely, if it rises to two teaspoons, you're venturing into diabetic territory with an associated risk of metabolic syndrome. Ideally, you'd want to maintain that "sweet spot" of just under one teaspoon.

Elevated glucose levels compel your body to amplify hormone regulation systems—boosting the release of insulin, cortisol, and adrenaline and potentially increasing fat tissue to help manage the surplus glucose.

For the first thirty days of the thyroid reboot, my default dietary template is 20 to 50 g of net carbohydrates (net carbs = carbs minus fiber). Going into month two, we can customize the carbohydrates according to stress, activity levels, and blood sugar sensitivity. The healthier your body responds to blood sugar, the more carbohydrates you can handle. The more out of balance your blood sugar becomes, or the more insulin resistance occurs, the more you have to be mindful of your carbohydrate intake. Insulin resistance increases your chance of developing metabolic syndrome, which comes with a whole host of issues ranging from high blood pressure to increased waist circumference and cardiovascular disease.

If you're entering this program at a relatively normal, healthy weight, within ten pounds or so of where you want to be, and your activity level is stable (e.g., exercising thirty minutes four times a week), you may be able to keep your carbohydrates at the higher end of that scale or even increase the maximum range to 75 or 150 g.

If weight gain is one of your top three chief complaints, your carbohydrate levels will start in the 20- to 50-gram range. Primarily, these carbohydrates will come from non-starchy vegetable sources, and maybe 10 to 20 percent of them will come from a low-sugar source, such as a low-sugar fruit (e.g., half a grapefruit, a green apple, one to two handfuls of berries, or a squeeze of lemon in your water).

Once we've assessed where you are, your diet plan is individualized based on your activity level and overall metabolic health. It's possible that we might even be able to add in some of the healthy starches (e.g., sweet potatoes, yams, squash, beets, or plantains). "The Meal Map" is one tool I created and use for my patients. It has columns for proteins, fats, carbs, and seasonings. The carbohydrates that are non-starchy are underlined. The carbohydrates that are starchy are starred. Lower-sugar fruits are italicized. Foods that are low in FODMAPs have (F) next to them; this pertains more to patients who have small intestinal bacterial overgrowth (SIBO). For any dietary template you choose, the Meal Map can be customized accordingly.

Of course, you can also find a link to download the PDF reference handout for the Meal Map in the resource section or at the end of the chapter.

Carbohydrate Levels

The carbohydrate levels in this section are provided in ranges of grams (g). These will give you some clues about where you should be. You will also learn the effects seen on the body at each level.

Ketosis and Fat Burning (0 to 50 g per day)

When you keep your carbohydrate intake near 50 g per day, you're going to enter a physiological state known as *ketosis lipolysis* or *nutritional ketosis*. Ketosis lipolysis is a normal state of physiology that involves primarily using fat for energy (this happens in fasting too). Fatty acids are broken down into ketone bodies. The body and brain then use these ketones for

THE MEAL MAP

PROTEINS		CARBS		FATS	SEASONINGS	
Bass	Snapper	Asparagus (F)	Lemon	Avocado (F)	Apple Cider Vinegar	
Bacon	Tilapia	Artichoke Heart (F)	Lime	Almonds	Allspice	Onion (F)
Buffalo	Turkey	Brussels Sprouts (F)	Lettuce	Butter	Bay Leaf	Pepper
Collagen	Tuna	Beets* (F)	Onions (F)	Bacon Fat	Basil	Paprika
Chicken Breast	Trout	Blackberries (F)	Peppers	Brazil Nuts	Curry	Rosemary
Chicken Thigh	Veal	Berries	Plantains*	Coconut Oil	Clove	Shallot (F)
Eggs	Venison	Bok Choy	Passion Fruit	Fish Oil	Cumin	Sea Salt
Flounder	Shrimp	Broccoli (F)	Sweet Potato*	Ghee	Cardamom	Thyme
Ground Beef		Collard Greens	Spinach	MCT Oil	Cinnamon	Tumeri
Halibut		Cabbage (F)	Squash*	Macadamia Oil	Chili Powder	
Lamb Chomps		Cucumber	Turnips*	Olive Oil	Celery Seed	
New York Steak		Chard	Tomatoes	Pecans	Dill	
Pea Protein		Celery	White Potato*	Seeds	Fenugreek	
Pork		Carrots	Yam*	Tallow	Ginger	
Ribs		Eggplant	Zucchini	Walnuts	Garlic (F)	
Rib Eye Steak		Green Beans			Garam Masala	
Salmon		Grape Fruit (F)			Herbs de Provence	
Sockeye		Green Apple (F)			Nutmeg	
Whey Protein		Kale			Oregano	

The Steps to Creating A Healthy Meal:

> AIP : Autoimmune
> Underline : Non-Starchy
> * : Safe Starch
> Italics : Low Sugar Fruit
> (F) : FODMAP

1. Pick your protein, carbs and fat.
2. Cook, sauté, grill or bake your protien.
3. Steam or saute your carbs with fat or eat raw.
4. Add herbs or seasoning to your dish for your flavor and variety.
5. Combine protein with carbs; if your protein is lean add additional fat to the meal.
6. Serve yourself a reasonable amount of food containing protein, fat and carbs.
7. If still hungry 5-10 minutes after your meal, continue with a second serving till comfortably full.
8. The meal should keep you full for at least 4-5 hours; if you are hungry sooner, you need to eat more.

fuel. Ketones also have an appetite-suppressing effect, and after a few weeks in ketosis, you will tend to lose your sweet cravings too.

The Sweet Spot! (50 to 100 g per day)

This is a spot I typically like to keep my carbohydrate range within; it allows me to not rely on exercise to stay lean and fit. If you have a damaged metabolism, a 0 to 50 g per day range may be where you need to live for a while. Some people also do well cycling in and out of ketosis: three or four days in a row in ketosis and one day in the sweet-spot range or higher. Carbohydrates are primarily used for instant energy, so if you're doing lots of exercise or you're under higher amounts of stress, getting a little bit of extra carbohydrates from healthy sources may be beneficial.

Maintenance (100 to 150 g per day)

Most people do well at maintaining their weight when their carbohydrates are within this range. Everyone is different, so depending on how damaged your metabolism is, this range may be too high for you. If you're relatively lean, exercise three to four times a week, and engage in activities like CrossFit, this will be a great place for you to be. I recommend timing a good chunk of your carbohydrate intake post-workout as a means to help improve recovery.

The Steady Track to Weight Gain (150 to 300 g per day)

When your carbohydrate levels are this high on a continuous basis, especially when there is no energy output to back it up, you are starting to push your body into an insulin-resistant state. The hormone that is secreted when you eat carbohydrates is insulin, and it primarily works by pulling carbohydrates and amino acids into your muscles. Like we talked about earlier, when your muscles and liver are saturated with carbohydrates, the rest of those carbohydrates will be stored as fat. When your carbohydrate intake is within the 150 to 300 g per day range, it's highly likely it will be stored as fat unless you are maintaining a consistent level of activity.

Danger, Will Robinson! (300 g or more per day)

If you're eating a diet based on the Food Guide Pyramid, it's more than likely that your carbohydrate intake will be in or around this range. All you have to do is eat a bagel every morning along with a glass of orange juice or bowl of cereal, have a sandwich for lunch with a Gatorade, and eat a plate of pasta for dinner, and you'll be on your way. Most people who are eating carbohydrates at this high level tend to have insulin resistance as well as increased risk markers for inflammation and metabolic syndrome. People who have a very high metabolism or are very active may be able to get away with this carb intake level.

Try Eating Your Carbohydrates at Night

Carb back-loading is a simple idea supported by some small studies. It suggests that eating most of your carbs in the evening might help with burning fat, controlling insulin, and reducing cravings. This method could be a useful addition to your diet plan. It's not a strict rule, but it's worth trying out.[2]

Cortisol levels are highest in the morning, and that cortisol allows your body to liberate stored glucose from your muscles and liver, which are easy to access. Glucose can also be created from protein (muscle tissues) or amino acids in your diet via gluconeogenesis.

Our body also converts a lot of energy from fats. So if you consume protein and fat in the morning, this primes your body to be a fat burner throughout the day. Protein-rich foods require a lot of energy for the body to break them down. Over 30 percent of the calories you take in from protein will be used in the digestion process of protein.[3] At night, your cortisol levels are the lowest, so providing extra carbs during this time frame can actually be beneficial. When cortisol is lower, like at night, your body's blood sugar levels can drop, which can cause your adrenals to make more adrenaline. A few more carbs at night in the form of some sweet potatoes or berries can help prevent these adrenaline spikes. Some may notice improved sleep because of this.

Thyroid Diet and Autoimmunity

Remember from Chapter 1 that in an autoimmune thyroid condition such as Hashimoto's, the immune system creates specific antibodies against itself. This causes immune cells to attack and destroy thyroid tissue and the ability of the thyroid gland to make thyroid hormone. Since 50 to 90 percent of thyroid issues are autoimmune in nature, it's important to cut out any foods that could stimulate an autoimmune reaction.[4] The big foods we want to cut out off the bat, for at least the first thirty days, are grains, legumes, dairy, nuts, seeds, eggs, and nightshades (tomatoes, potatoes, eggplants, and peppers).

With the percentage of autoimmunity in thyroid issues being so high, we have to make sure you aren't eating foods that could potentially exacerbate the autoimmune condition. You really want to set yourself up for success. So for the first thirty days, eliminating all autoimmune-provoking foods is going to be the best way to go because when you start adding foods—nuts, seeds, nightshades, legumes, and so on—back in after that first month, if the body reacts, you're going to notice it.

Dietary Tips

To help you balance blood sugar, optimize hormone levels, minimize adrenal fatigue, prevent ups and downs in energy and mood, improve autoimmune conditions, and promote weight loss, you need to know how to eat and what to eat. The following lists are from my "Just In Health Eating Plan." I also have a reference handout that you are welcome to download and print, found in the resources section.

Functional Glucose Tolerance Testing

A reliable way to determine your insulin resistance is by examining your blood sugar levels. Monitoring your blood sugar just before eating and for three to four hours afterward can reveal how insulin-resistant you are. The longer and higher your blood sugar remains elevated, the more insulin your pancreas produces to lower it.

Blood sugar can rise due to inflammatory foods and an excess of carbohydrates. Inflammatory foods can trigger cortisol and adrenaline, causing a stress response. These stress hormones mobilize glucose to help cope with stress. However, if the glucose isn't used, it's often stored as fat, contributing to weight gain and other health issues.

Carbohydrates are broken down into glucose in your bloodstream. Consuming a high amount of carbs, particularly from sources like processed flour, grains, and foods containing high-fructose corn syrup, can lead to significant increases in your blood glucose levels. Fruits with high fructose content, such as tropical fruits, are the next most impactful. Safer starches, like sweet potatoes or white potatoes, which are primarily glucose-based, have a lesser effect on blood sugar levels. Non-starchy vegetables like leafy greens have the lowest impact on your blood sugar and provide significant micronutrients like potassium and magnesium.

Choosing to eat whole foods, like fruits or safer starches, provides numerous benefits. These foods contain fiber, which helps release sugar more gradually into your bloodstream, preventing rapid blood sugar spikes. Conversely, processed foods like flour-based products or junk food with added sugar are absorbed more quickly, causing blood sugar levels to rise rapidly.

To better understand how various foods impact your blood sugar, you can perform a functional glucose tolerance test. This test involves measuring your blood sugar before and after consuming different types of foods, allowing you to see how your body responds to each. By analyzing the results, you can make informed dietary choices that help manage your blood sugar levels and reduce insulin resistance, ultimately improving your overall health.

> **Point of clarity**: A functional glucose tolerance test is different than a glucose tolerance test, which typically gives an individual 75 g of glucose in a drink, then tests their blood sugar after. This test is a functional test as it uses your typical meal instead.

Step 1

Measure your glucose levels upon waking up or just before eating a meal. Keep in mind that in the early morning, a cortisol spike known as the dawn phenomenon can raise your blood sugar levels independently of your diet. This is why we want to check other meals throughout the day as well.

Step 2

Monitor your blood sugar at one, two, three, and four hours after eating. Aim for the following ranges:

- One hour: 120–140 (or lower)
- Two hours: 100–120 (or lower)
- Three hours: less than 100 (ideally 80–95)
- Four hours: test only if your blood sugar is still above 100 in hour three

Step 3

If your blood sugar is outside the target range, try light exercises such as walking, air squats, or jumping jacks to lower it. After a meal, opt for a gentle five- to ten-minute walk. If you notice consistently elevated blood sugar, record the carbs consumed in the problematic meal and reduce them for the next meal.

Step 4

Test your blood sugar levels during three different meals (e.g., breakfast, lunch, or dinner) throughout the week. Cortisol fluctuations can impact blood sugar, so testing at various times helps identify any changes in your readings.

Step 5

Improve your body's glucose management by incorporating nutrients like chromium, magnesium, B vitamins, vanadium, cinnamon, gymnema, myoinositol, and alpha-lipoic acid. Prioritize dietary changes, then lifestyle modifications like exercise, and finally consider supplements. This approach will help you determine if you need to adjust your carbohydrate intake.

Consider using a *continuous glucose monitor* (CGM), such as the FreeStyle Libre or Dexcom. These devices attach to your arm and connect to a smartphone app, providing a visual representation of your blood sugar levels on a graph. Sometimes CGMs can be inaccurate, so it's essential to compare their readings with a traditional finger prick test if necessary. Some CGMs, like the Dexcom, can be calibrated for increased accuracy.

If you're not comfortable using a continuous glucose monitor, there are other options available. You could try the same procedure that people with type 1 diabetes use, which is a traditional finger-prick test for blood sugar. You can find reliable testing kits at your local drugstore, and we will provide some links in the resources section at the end of this book. Another option is to use a blood sugar meter like the Keto-Mojo, which not only measures blood glucose but also ketone levels. Ketone levels are a good indicator of whether your carb intake is low enough to enter a state of fat burning. Ideally, a ketone reading between 0.5 and 3 millimoles per liter is optimal. A fasting insulin blood test is another good marker to test; ideally below 7 µIU/mL is good sign you aren't insulin resistant.

HOW TO EAT

1. **Eat Every Four to Five Hours:** This relieves your adrenal glands from the job of maintaining normal blood sugar levels between meals via adrenaline and cortisol. If you are waiting until you're hungry, it's too late. If you can't last four to five hours, you probably aren't eating enough protein and fat.

2. **Eat Real Food:** Eat real foods, ideally three times more veggies than fruit. If you are currently overweight, you may need to remove fruit and starch from your diet until you become leaner and healthier. Please avoid fruit juices; they can be very high in sugar.

3. **Combine Protein, Fat, and Carbs**: Always combine protein, fat, and carbohydrates together. It is important you consume 30 g of protein in the first thirty minutes of waking for breakfast. A fist size of animal protein is roughly 30 g of protein or about 4 oz.

   a. Animal Protein Amounts: one palm or fist to one full hand; this equals 3 to 8 ounces per meal.

   b. Carbohydrate Amounts: two fists to two full hands. Half to three-quarters of your plate should be veggies per meal.

   c. Use the Meal Map to create your meals; carbs are optional in the morning unless you're eating veggies.

4. **Dial In Your Carbs**: Most people do well starting off on a lower carb diet of 50 g or less. As your metabolism heals, you may be able to increase your carbs.

   a. Carbs below 50 g: great for insulin resistance, weight gain, and a damaged metabolism.

   b. Carbs 50-100 g: up your carbs to this level if you experience fatigue and weight gain with lower carbs; increasing carbs may help. It may be normal to feel a little fatigue the first week or so as your body is converting to a new primary fuel source, fat.

    c. Carbs 100–150+ g: stay at this level if you are exercising more, feeling good, and happy with your weight.

5. **Reduce Inflammation**: The foods recommended are anti-inflammatory, nutrient dense, and low in toxins. They provide building blocks to help heal your hormones, your brain, and your energy systems. Every bite of food is either promoting inflammation or healing. The choice is yours!

6. **Minimize Stimulants**: Caffeine stimulants like coffee or tea work by provoking the stress-handling glands into releasing epinephrine and cortisol to raise blood sugar and release energy. If you consume them, make it organic and add fats like MCT oil, butter, ghee, and/or collagen amino acids if tolerated.

7. **Use Sea Salt**: Your adrenal glands need adequate amounts of sea salt and trace minerals for healthy function, especially if you have low blood pressure and get dizzy when changing body position. Favorite brands: Real Salt, Himalayan sea salt, and Celtic Sea Salt.

    a. Take up to one-half teaspoon of sea salt two times per day for symptoms of low minerals, including dizziness upon rising and low blood pressure. You can also salt your food liberally at each meal.

8. **Drink Plenty of Clean Water**: You should be drinking half your body weight in ounces. If you weigh 200 pounds, that's 100 ounces of water. Use water that is filtered or a reliable spring water source, not tap water. Do not drink water with food; wait ten to fifteen minutes before or at least two hours after a meal to prevent diluted digestive juices and enzymes.

WHAT TO EAT

1. **Eat Omega-3 Fats**: Eat foods rich in omega-3's like fatty cold-water fish, including salmon, tuna, trout, herring, and mackerel. Or, if you prefer, take an omega-3 supplement. Please see your health care provider for recommendations. Avoid fish that are high in mercury like shark and swordfish and oil. Eat fish that are wild, not farmed.

2. **Eat Healthy Saturated and Monounsaturated Fats**: Coconut oil, ghee, MCT oil, grass-fed butter, tallow, and extra virgin olive oil. Note: Avoid canola oil and soy oil which are highly refined and genetically engineered, and have none of the benefits of the oils mentioned.

3. **Eat Healthy Carbs:** Eat six to eight or more servings of organic vegetables and fruits every day. It is important that you consume two to three times more vegetables than fruit. Fruits should be minimized until your weight loss goal is achieved. Vegetables and fruits should be fresh or frozen, not canned. Vegetables can be eaten raw if your digestion is well; if not, then steam, sauté, or consume your veggies in soup or stew form.

4. **Eat Healthy Proteins:** Pasture fed and preferably organic or at least free-range animal products.

5. **Meats:** Fish, chicken, beef, eggs, lamb, venison, or pork are great sources.

6. **The Paleo Template:** No grains, legumes, or dairy (focus on healthy amounts of fats, protein, and carbs).
   a. Grains: Wheat, barley, rye, rice, spelt, kamut, oat, corn, quinoa, and amaranth.
   b. Legumes: Beans, lentils, peanuts, and soy.
   c. Dairy: Milk, yogurt, and cheese. Grass-fed butter and ghee may be OK if tolerated.

7. **The Autoimmune Template:** For more serious cases, an Autoimmune Template may be needed. Remove grains, legumes, dairy, nuts, seeds, nightshade

vegetables (tomatoes, potatoes, eggplant, and peppers), and eggs. Remember to rotate your proteins and vegetables to avoid creating food allergies for foods that are consumed more frequently. FODMAPs may need to be removed if constipation, bloating, or gas doesn't improve in the first month. Avoid eating raw foods if you have active digestive issues.

8. **Be Diligent**: The unhealthier and more inflamed you are, the more diligent you need to be in adhering to the dietary guidelines set forward. When it comes time to add more foods back in, please refer to the link in the resources section to see the "Diet Reintroduction Handout." Please wait at least four weeks and until you have plateaued for one week on the diet before adding in new foods.

9. **Artificial Sweeteners**: Avoid artificial sweeteners like Splenda and aspartame. Healthier sweetener options include monk fruit and stevia in moderation. See the recommended products linked at the end of the chapter.

10. **No Gluten-Free Junk Food**: These foods tend to be higher in sugar and often contain other refined grains. Most gluten-free grains can still cause problems for individuals with gluten sensitivity.

11. **Recommended Products**: The list includes high-quality snacks, air filters, water filters, and devices that can improve your health.

12. **Use the Meal Map**: There are literally thousands of potential meal options or combinations if you use the Meal Map. If you are becoming bored with your food, you need to start mixing things up.

Dietary Tools

There are many dietary tools you can utilize to keep track of your progress on the thyroid reboot diet. You can plug your foods in and get a macronutrient breakdown of how much you are consuming and what your percentage is for each. The nutrient counter app will also give you a micronutrient and macronutrient breakdown, which is great to see if you are getting enough magnesium or potassium. To access the nutrient counter, see the resources section.

You can easily use apps like this to share your nutrition information with your functional medicine practitioner to help monitor your progress. Are your macronutrients good? Are you eating a good amount of fats? How's your protein consumption based on your activity, height, and weight? Are the carbohydrate levels at a good place? Your practitioner can also look at the quality of your food choices and advise you based on what you input into the app.

If you prefer the paper route, you can use a diet diary that records your meals, mealtimes, bedtimes, and so on, and share it with your practitioner at each visit. There is a reference handout for the "Diet Diary" I give my patients, which you can find in the resources section.

Exercise

Exercise can increase your energy and make you feel good when done properly. But it can be a physical stressor (remember the Triangle of Health from Chapter 1) and wreak havoc on your body when it's overdone or not done correctly.

There are three questions you need to be able to answer yes to in order to make sure you're exercising correctly.

1. Is the exercise energizing me, and do I feel good after the exercise?
2. About ten to fifteen minutes after I finish exercising, do I emotionally feel I could repeat the exercise?
3. Do I feel good later that day and/or the next morning? Or do I feel overly tired and sore?

Do you finish your exercise and think, *I'm done—I just don't have one more ounce of energy in me*? Do you feel that runner's high but know there's no way you could possibly repeat the exercise that day or the next morning? Do you feel like a bus hit you? If so, your exercise frequency, intensity, or duration need to be adjusted. It may be normal to feel sore after doing newer movements, but if you're doing things that are relatively the same or similar, your body shouldn't feel that run down.

Exercise's Effect on Metabolism

If you're doing lots of long-distance aerobic exercises, such as your typical marathon or distance running, the research is very clear that this type of exercise stimulates cortisol and actually lowers your metabolism. The reason it lowers your metabolism is because your body is designed to be as efficient as possible when exercising. When you're running, your body is actually trying to get more energy done with fewer calories (i.e., lowering your metabolism).

When you exercise, you want your body to be incredibly inefficient when it comes to burning fuel. This is because you want the fuel your body is burning to come from fat. When the body is inefficient at burning fuel, meaning it's burning a lot more than normal, this will boost your metabolism. It's also important to choose the right kinds of exercises that aid this process—ideally resistance training, where you're doing movements that involve moving weights, or functional full-body movements (squatting, lunging, etc.) that will stimulate your muscles to grow. The more muscle mass you have, the more storage for extra carbs you will also have. Muscles are naturally more metabolically active, so they will also consume more calories while your body is at rest.

What Is the Best Exercise?

High-intensity interval training—bursts of high-intensity exercise followed by periods of rest and relaxation—is great for metabolism because it stimulates a hormone called *human growth hormone* (HGH).

HGH increases metabolism and helps you put on muscle for up to twenty-four hours after the movement is completed.[5] This is the big advantage to doing resistance training and high-intensity interval training. High-intensity sprints or biking, for example, for thirty seconds, followed by a sixty- to ninety-second rest or relaxation period, can be incredibly powerful because your metabolism after ten to thirty minutes of that movement is now increased for up to twenty-four hours afterward. This phenomenon is known as *EPOC* (excess post-exercise oxygen consumption), and it has a long-lasting impact on your metabolism compared to any other exercise. That out-of-breath feeling after exercise is a good sign you are experiencing EPOC.

The main metabolic benefit that you get from aerobic training happens only while you're doing the movement, so you don't get that major metabolic increase after a long-distance, steady aerobic session. Aerobic exercise tends to be more cortisol stimulating, so if you already have adrenal fatigue issues, and your cortisol is already out of balance, continuing with more aerobic exercise is actually going to beat down your adrenal glands. The adrenals are really important for thyroid health, as you will see when we get to the adrenal chapter.

Zone 2 cardio is a type of low-impact workout known for its benefits in enhancing mitochondrial function and promoting fat loss. This exercise can be performed on a bike, rower, elliptical, or treadmill for a duration of thirty to forty-five minutes. The objective is to maintain your heart rate in the lower 100s, aiming for a pace where you can comfortably hold a conversation without gasping for breath, yet it's evident to others that you're engaging in physical activity.

Sleep

We all know that feeling of waking up from a really good night of sleep when you feel like a brand-new person. But unfortunately, we also know the feeling of waking up to that alarm and asking ourselves, *Did I even sleep?* When we have restful, restorative sleep, we are able to pass through all four stages of sleep five times throughout the night. One of these stages is rapid eye movement (REM), when your body repairs and heals. It takes about ninety minutes to go through one complete sleep cycle, where all four stages of sleep are achieved.

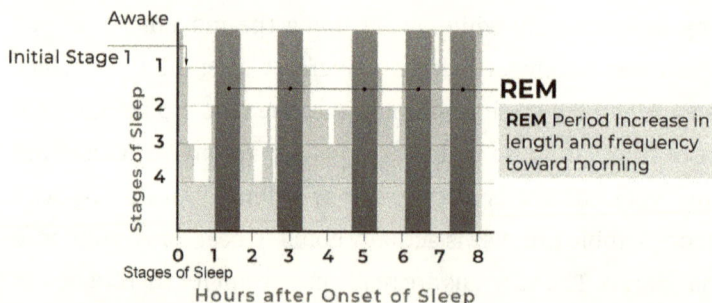

REM
REM Period Increase in length and frequency toward morning

Hours after Onset of Sleep

The body is naturally programmed to repair physiologically and structurally between the hours of 10:00 p.m. and 2:00 a.m., when you are healing and your repairing growth hormone peaks. If you're not getting to bed on time, you're limiting your ability to tap into that needed growth hormone. When you are stressed and inflamed, your body needs that repair, so the sooner you can get to bed, the more you're able to build muscle and help your body heal.[6]

Muscle is the most metabolically active tissue in the body, so the more muscle you have, the more you're going to be able to burn fat for energy while resting, and the more reserves you'll have for carbohydrates and sugars. People who tend to handle carbohydrates better are the ones who have more muscle because the extra carbohydrates can be put into your muscle cells for fuel rather than putting them into fat cells for storage. Extra carbohydrates and sugars always get thrown into fat cells if there is no room in the muscles or the liver for them. The more extra muscle you have, the more your metabolism can burn it up, and the more your muscle can act as a reservoir for storage.

Muscle is like a sponge for glucose or sugar. The more muscle you have, the more it acts like wringing out a sponge. Once the sponge is wrung out, it has more ability to absorb liquid, or in this case, glucose. A sponge that is not wrung out adequately loses its ability to absorb water, or in this case, sugar and glucose. So the next time you are exercising, imagine you're wringing out a sponge. Healing and restorative sleep during the optimal hours helps build this muscle.

The Circadian Rhythm—the Body's Natural Clock

The circadian rhythm is the body's natural clock based on light and dark cycles. Humans have this beautiful rhythm: when the sun comes up in the morning, this stimulates cortisol, a hormone that tells the body it's time to get up. When the sun goes down and darkness sets in, this drives down cortisol and stimulates melatonin, a hormone that tells the body it's time to sleep.

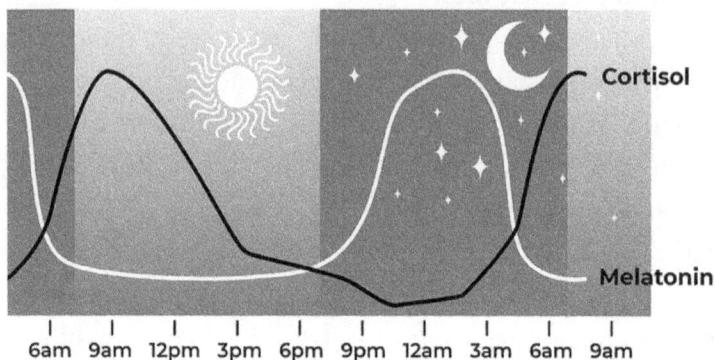

There have been many studies done on the circadian rhythms of shift workers. According to an article regarding night workers in the *Monitor on Psychology*, "Millions of American workers fight against their circadian clocks every day," and even with plenty of sleep during other hours, "all the sleep in the world won't make up for circadian misalignment."[7]

The World Health Organization (WHO), through its component agency, the International Agency for Research on Cancer (IARC), has actually found that lack of sleep is the only non-substance carcinogen known to man; it's in the same category as asbestos and smoking.[8] Shift workers have an increased risk for all-cause mortality, especially cancer and heart disease.

Sleep deprivation also disrupts the body's circadian rhythm and can lead to an imbalance in blood sugar, insulin issues, and thyroid problems. So getting enough sleep and getting it during the right hours is vital.

The Earlier You Go to Bed, the Better

The lowering of cortisol and stimulation of melatonin peaks between 10:00 p.m. and 12:00 a.m., when neurological and structural repair happen. This is why, physically, healing and restorative sleep are most beneficial during those hours.

The body also repairs psychologically during sleep, and this happens between 2:00 a.m. and 6:00 a.m. So if you get to bed at 3:00 a.m., you may still be able to function mentally, but your body may not feel very good.

Tips for Getting Good Sleep

There are many things we do at night, especially in today's technology-driven world, that can throw off your melatonin production and keep your cortisol levels artificially high. This list of sleeping tips will help you establish the right nighttime conditions that will allow you to go to sleep on time and stay asleep:

1. Turn off all electronic devices (TVs, computers, tablets, etc.) at least one hour before bed. The blue light in these devices suppresses melatonin. Melatonin is a hormone that is primarily useful for restoration and helps you sleep.

2. If you must use electronic devices after 8:00 p.m., use blue-blocking sunglasses. There's also an app for your computer called f.lux (justgetflux.com) that can help block blue light. Make sure your phone is in airplane mode and keep it at least six feet away from you when you go to sleep to avoid any EMF radiating from your device.

3. Use dimmers or keep the lights low in your house before bedtime. Bright lights can slow the production of melatonin.

4. Make sure your bedroom is completely dark at night. Lights from clocks, phones, nightlights, and so on, as well as lights coming in through the windows, can disrupt your body's rhythm. If you can see your hand in front of your face when you turn out your light, it's not dark enough.

KEY POINTS

1. Maintaining a proper diet is one of the most important things you can do to keep your thyroid healthy. Please be aware of the other thyroid connections that impact thyroid function (gut, female/male hormones, adrenal, detox, and infections).

2. Three main criteria form the foundation of the thyroid reboot nutrition plan: food must be nutrient dense, anti-inflammatory, and low in toxins.

3. Consume a healthy balance of macronutrients— proteins, fats, and carbohydrates.

4. High blood sugar or insulin resistance will keep your body from metabolically activating and converting your thyroid hormone.

5. High-intensity interval exercise and restorative sleep that balances your circadian rhythm are two important things you can do to positively impact your thyroid health.

Resources

Thyroid Reboot Foundations Bundle (www.justinhealth. com/foundations) Here are several recommended thyroid-supporting supplements mentioned in the book in easy-to-access bundles.

Meal Map Diet Handout (www.justinhealth.com/meal-map) This is the quick-start diet guide that I use with my patients. There are some simple diet and lifestyle strategies laid out here that are easy to follow.

Whole House Filtration (www.justinhealth.com/water-filters) This is a recommendation for the whole-house filter I use in my own home. This filter is carbon-based and has a pre- and post-filter for larger sediments as well.

Water Filtration Reverse Osmosis (www.justinhealth.com/ reverse-osmosis) Here you can find an under-the-counter reverse osmosis filter that I personally endorse. Reverse osmosis has the highest level of filtration.

Water Pitcher Gravity Filter (www.justinhealth.com/water-pitcher) Here is a more affordable water filter option, especially if you can't modify the house you live in for a water filter installation. This water pitcher filters out far more toxins than your typical gravity water pitcher filter.

Micronutrients and Macronutrient Counter (www. justinhealth.com/nutrient-counter) This is a nutrient counter that will track your macronutrients like protein, fat, carbs, and overall calories, which is standard for an app like this. What's different about this one is that it will also look at micronutrients like magnesium, potassium, etc.

Dexcom Blood Sugar Meter (www.justinhealth.com/dexcom) This is a continuous blood glucose monitor; you may need a doctor's prescription to access it.

FreeStyle Libre (www.justinhealth.com/libre) This is a continuous blood glucose monitor; you may need a doctor's prescription to access it.

Keto-Mojo Ketone and Blood Sugar Meter (www. justinhealth.com/ketomojo) This is an excellent blood sugar meter that will connect to your phone via Bluetooth and graph your blood sugar levels. It can also test for ketones.

Blue Blocking Glasses (www.justinhealth.com/glasses) These glasses are independently lab-tested to guarantee a blue light reduction of 99 percent or more.

Diet Reintroduction Handout (http://www.justinhealth.com/ diet-reintroduction) This handout instructs you how to add foods back into your diet.

Recommended Products (www.justinhealth.com/approved-products) This list includes high-quality snacks, air filters, water filters, and devices that can improve your health.

Notes

1   Stephan Guyenet, "By 2606, the US Diet Will Be 100 Percent Sugar," *Whole Health Source: Nutrition and Health* Science (blog), February 18, 2012, https://wholehealthsource.blogspot. com/2012/02/by-2606-us-diet-will-be-100-percent.html.

2   Amber W. Kinsey and Michael J. Ormsbee, "The Health Impact of Nighttime Eating: Old and New Perspectives," *Nutrients* 7, no. 4 (2015): 2648–62, https://doi.org/10.3390/nu7042648; and Eunho Chun et al., "Alleviation of Irritable Bowel Syndrome-Like Symptoms and Control of Gut and Brain Responses with Oral Administration of *Dolichos Iablab* L. in a Mouse Model," *Nutrients* 10, no. 10 (2018): 1475, https://doi.org/10.3390/nu10101475.

3   Dominik H. Pesta and Varman T. Samuel, "A High-Protein Diet for Reducing Body Fat: Mechanisms and Possible Caveats," *Nutrition & Metabolism* 11 (2014): 53, https://doi.org/10.1186/1743-7075-11-53.

4   Amino, "Autoimmunity and Hypothyroidism."

5   Beau Kjerulf Greer et al., "Comparison between Resistance Training and High-Intensity Interval Training in Aerobically Fit Women," *International Journal of Exercise* 14, no. 2 (2021): 1027–35, https://www.ncbi.nlm.nih.gov/pmc/articles/PMC8439678.

6   J. R. Davidson, H. Moldofsky, and F. A. Lue, "Growth Hormone and Cortisol Secretion in Relation to Sleep and Wakefulness," *Journal of Psychiatry and Neuroscience* 16, no. 2 (July 1991): 96–102, https:// www.ncbi.nlm.nih.gov/pmc/articles/PMC1188300.

7   Michael Price, "The Risks of Night Work," *Monitor on Psychology* 42, no. 1 (January 2011): 38, https://www.apa.org/monitor/2011/01/ night-work.

8   "Rotating Night Shift Work Can Be Hazardous to Your Health," Science News, Science Daily, January 5, 2015, https://www. sciencedaily.com/releases/2015/01/150105081757.htm.

3

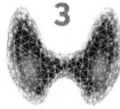

The Gut Connection

WHAT HAPPENS IN THE GUT DOESN'T STAY IN the gut! All the nutrients that make your thyroid hormone are absorbed in the gut. The health of your gastrointestinal system impacts every system in your body, including your immune system, detoxification system, circulatory system, and others. This is why the gut connection is so important.

Did you know 80 percent of all your immune cells live in your GALT (*gastric associated lymphoid tissue*) in your stomach or your MALT (*mucosa associated lymphoid tissue*) in your small intestines? The likelihood that your immune system will malfunction and attack your thyroid gland via an autoimmune response (think Hashimoto's) increases as digestive stress and inflammation have a greater impact on it.[1]

Remember, you have T4 and T3 thyroid hormones, and T4 is your inactive hormone, while T3 is your active hormone. The enzyme that actually breaks down T4 to T3 (deiodinase) is a selenium-based enzyme. So not only iodine, but also healthy levels of selenium are needed to make this thyroid conversion from inactive to active thyroid hormone. Without healthy gut function and a nutrient-dense diet, there may not be enough building blocks to make this conversion happen.

The Importance of Stomach Acid

In Chapter 1, you learned about the Triangle of Health and the Triple-S Approach (stressors, systems, symptoms). One of the big systems on that second S (body systems) is the *gastrointestinal* (GI) system. When the GI system starts becoming stressed, low stomach acid, or *hydrochloric acid* (HCl), results. Stomach acid is necessary to lower the pH in the stomach. With enough healthy stomach acid, the following domino effect in the first steps of digestion begins:

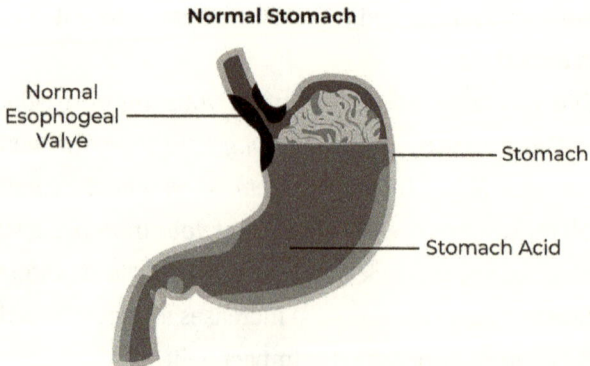

Normal Stomach

Normal Esophogeal Valve

Stomach

Stomach Acid

1. Healthy stomach acid lowers the pH.
   a. Low pH activates *proteolytic enzymes* (*pepsin*), which break down protein.
   b. The broken-down food is called chyme, and chyme needs to ideally measure around a 2 or 3 on the pH scale.

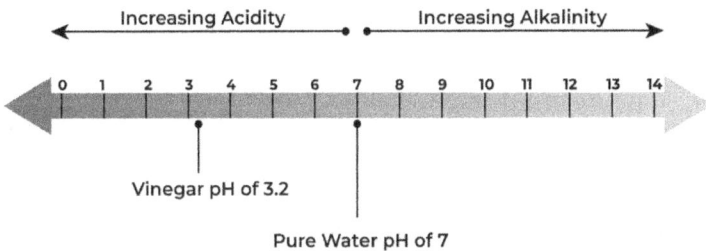

Increasing Acidity   Increasing Alkalinity

| 0 | 1 | 2 | 3 | 4 | 5 | 6 | 7 | 8 | 9 | 10 | 11 | 12 | 13 | 14 |

Vinegar pH of 3.2

Pure Water pH of 7

2. The acidic chyme gets released into your small intestine and triggers your gallbladder to produce bile via a hormone called cholecystokinin (CCK). The pancreas is also triggered to produce lipase, trypsin, and chymotrypsin (proteolytic and lipolytic enzymes) to aid in protein and fat digestion.

3. Bile and lipase help break down and emulsify fat, kind of like how Dawn dish soap breaks down fat on a greasy pan. Trypsin and chymotrypsin help break down proteins.

The Effects of Stress on the Gut

Managing and adapting to stress is important because it is part of a healthy nervous system. Imagine that the nervous system has only a gas pedal and a brake pedal, just like your car. The *parasympathetic nervous system*, like the brake, is the slow-down, rest, and digest part of the nervous system. The *sympathetic nervous system* is the go-go-go, accelerate part of the nervous system.[2]

When your parasympathetic nervous system is turned on, you're resting, relaxing, meditating, going for a walk, or having an engaging conversation. When your sympathetic nervous system is turned on it causes different types of stress, like eating inflammatory foods, fighting with your spouse, and so on.

You drive a car with only one foot—your right foot. Your right foot can't be on the gas and the brake at the same time. So you're either hitting the gas pedal (sympathetic nervous system), which means you're feeling stressed, or you're hitting the brake pedal (parasympathetic nervous system), which means you're slowing down, resting, repairing, and being mindful.

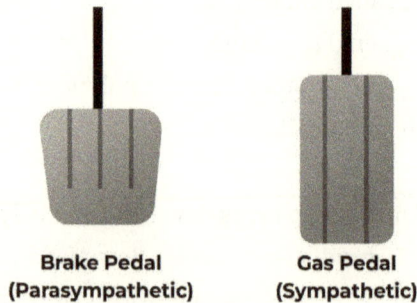

**Brake Pedal
(Parasympathetic)**   **Gas Pedal
(Sympathetic)**

When the sympathetic nervous system is overactivated, stomach acid will be lower, as that requires energy. The more stressed you are, the more you're hitting the gas pedal and the more you're turning off digestion. The stress hormones cortisol and adrenaline are pumping to mobilize glucose, so your arms and legs have an energy source so they can run, fight, and flee. Your body is hardwired to allocate survival as a top priority. When you're in survival mode, the need to feel hunger or digest food gets scrapped as a secondary priority.

The hydrochloric acid (HCl) in the stomach also keeps the bad microbes from accumulating, lowers the pH, and helps activate your enzymes. It keeps the gut cleaner and makes it harder for outside invaders to grow.[3]

Peristalsis

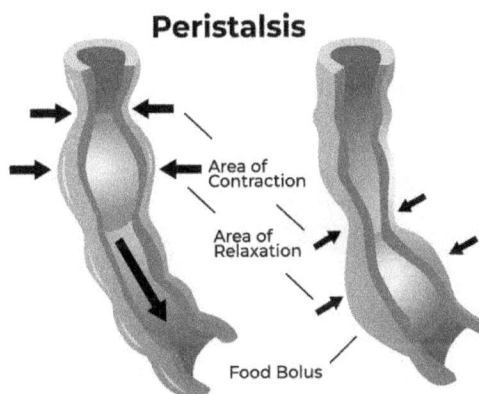

Area of Contraction

Area of Relaxation

Food Bolus

Disruption of Peristalsis

Peristalsis is the wavelike contraction in the intestines that helps move stool out. Think of peristalsis as the process of getting toothpaste out of a toothpaste tube. You have to roll the tube to get the toothpaste out. Thyroid hormone is instrumental in helping to create peristalsis, and one of the big things seen in hypothyroidism (low thyroid hormone) is constipation.[4]

Relief of constipation is a common thing that can occur when someone is given thyroid hormone because the hormone helps aid in peristalsis. If someone's constipation doesn't improve, it could be due to other gut infections creating stress in the digestive tract.

Anemia

Anemia just means a lack of healthy red blood cells. In B_{12} deficiency, there's what's known as *macrocytic anemia*, when the blood cells stay really big and goofy. As red blood cells get older, more mature, and refined, they should actually get smaller. If you have an iron deficiency, this is known as *microcytic anemia*. The red blood cells get too small.

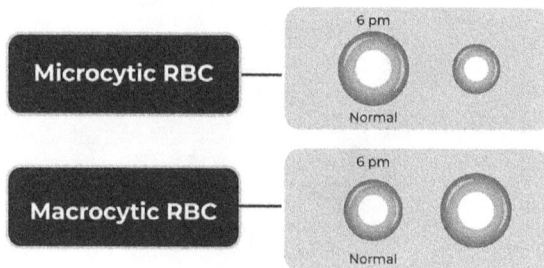

Stomach acid breaks down and ionizes minerals, such as iron and selenium. This basically means it turns them into a form in which the body can take them up, absorb them, and bring them into the bloodstream. If stomach acid is low, minerals cannot properly be ionized. It is comparable to sand on a street that a solid asphalt surface will never be able to absorb. Rather than absorbing minerals, many may move right through the body.

B$_{12}$ Deficiency (Macrocytic Anemia)

Another condition that poor digestion exacerbates is B$_{12}$ deficiency. B$_{12}$ is needed to make healthy red blood cells. Red blood cells are needed to carry nutrition and oxygen throughout the body, which fuels metabolism. Think back to middle school science class when you had to place a glass jar over a candle. Within a few seconds, that candle went out because it needed oxygen for metabolic fuel. Without oxygen, the candle can't stay lit. With a deficiency in B$_{12}$, red blood cells can't function optimally, and the body's ability to carry oxygen and nutrition will be impaired. This will affect energy levels, mitochondrial function, and thyroid hormone levels.

According to some studies, as many as 28 percent of Hashimoto's patients have B$_{12}$ deficiency, and of those with a B$_{12}$ deficiency, 31 percent also have pernicious anemia.[5] This is when the parietal cells in your stomach produce B$_{12}$. The compound that absorbs B$_{12}$ is called *intrinsic factor*. The parietal cells produce an intrinsic factor that helps bind to the B$_{12}$ in foods you eat. The immune system—especially if you have autoimmune disorders—will attack either the parietal cell (parietal cell antibodies), rendering the cell unable to make intrinsic factor, or it will attack the intrinsic factor (intrinsic factor antibodies) made by the cell, making the B$_{12}$ difficult to absorb in the small intestine.[6]

Autoimmunity is the major reason your gut may have a difficult time absorbing B$_{12}$. The immune system that is interfering with B$_{12}$ absorption is the same immune system that could be attacking your thyroid too. This is why it's so important to address the underlying immune stressors that are damaging your thyroid, either directly in the case of Hashimoto's or indirectly in the case of B_{12} deficiency.

B_{12} is found in high amounts in quality animal products like beef, chicken, liver, and pork. If you are a vegan or vegetarian, you could be at a major risk for B_{12} deficiency if you are not already supplementing B_{12}.

Iron Deficiency (Microcytic Anemia)

Iron is part of the hemoglobin protein molecule, which helps carry oxygen to your tissues. Iron is also another building block in the thyroid hormone cascade.[7] You learned about tyrosine, iodine, and selenium, but there are some background nutrients that are also important for that thyroid-building process, and iron is one of these background nutrients. Iron is another one of those nutrients that is abundant in animal products. You can find nonheme iron in leafy greens like spinach, which is less absorbable due to anti-nutrients in plants, like phytates and oxalates.[8] Heme iron from animal products does not have these additional anti-nutrients attached to it, which makes it more soluble and easier to absorb.

Zinc Deficiency

Zinc is a building block for stomach acid.[9] With low stomach acid, you can't break down zinc. Zinc is also needed to *make* more stomach acid, so if you can't break down zinc, you create a larger deficiency, and the initial low-stomach-acid problem actually gets worse and worse, like a downward spiral. Zinc is an important building block for the thyroid because without it, stomach acid can't be made. And if you can't make stomach acid, you can't ionize and absorb all the nutrients needed for healthy thyroid function. Zinc also help thickens the gastric mucosa making it more resistant against acid levels.[10]

Additional Deficiencies

In addition to iron, B_{12}, zinc, iodine, and selenium (which were covered in Chapter 1), there are other mineral and vitamin deficiencies that can impacted by gut stress and affect thyroid function. They include the following:

- Magnesium
- Calcium
- Copper
- Chromium

- Vitamin A
- Vitamin D
- Vitamin E
- Vitamin K

Gut Bacteria and the Thyroid

Keeping bad gut bacteria in balance is imperative for a healthy gut and thyroid health. It's so important that an entire chapter, "The Infection Connection," is dedicated to it later in this book. But for reference purposes, there are a few things about bacteria that need to be addressed here as well.

A healthy gut microbiome consists of over 100 trillion microbes of bacteria, viruses, and fungus, weighing almost five pounds! The microbiome is collectively known as the "second human genome" and is now referred to as a separate organ.[11] I know, right? It is crazy to think about. However, the majority of the bacteria should be beneficial, good bacteria, with a much smaller percentage of dysbiosis, or bad bacteria. When these numbers start to skew in the other direction and more bad bacteria than good bacteria start to occur, we call this *dysbiosis*.

There are generally two types of aerobic bacteria in the gut: gram-negative and gram-positive. *Gram-negative bacteria* have two membranes, or two walls, and *gram-positive bacteria* have one. Gram-positive bacteria are like a house that has a door to enter (one barrier, or one wall). Gram-negative bacteria are like a castle that has a moat and a steep wall to go through (two barriers, or two walls) to enter.

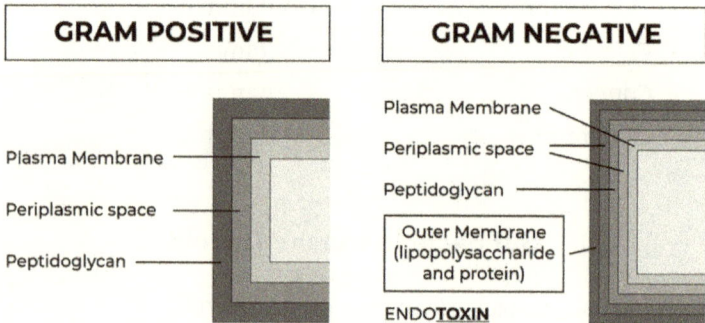

GRAM POSITIVE

Plasma Membrane
Periplasmic space
Peptidoglycan

GRAM NEGATIVE

Plasma Membrane
Periplasmic space
Peptidoglycan
Outer Membrane (lipopolysaccharide and protein)
ENDOTOXIN

What this means is that those gram-negative bacteria are harder to kill because they have cell walls. This makes it more difficult for an antibiotic or an herbal antibiotic protocol to penetrate and eradicate the microbes. The greater the microbial load, the increased chance you may experience side effects due to a die-off reaction or a *Herxheimer reaction*. These die-off symptoms (fatigue, brain fog, achiness, bloating, gas, constipation, or diarrhea) are due to the outer wall of the bacteria containing an endotoxin or lipopolysaccharide (LPS), which can be hard on the detoxification system.

What Is Helicobacter pylori (H. pylori)?

Helicobacter pylori (*H. pylori*) is a particularly stubborn gram-negative bacteria shaped like a helix, which is where it gets its name. Gram-negative bacteria like H. pylori can be difficult to eradicate due to a feature known as an *efflux pump*. Efflux pumps work by pumping the antimicrobial herbs or antibiotic medications right out of the bacteria's cell wall, making it much harder to kill.[12]

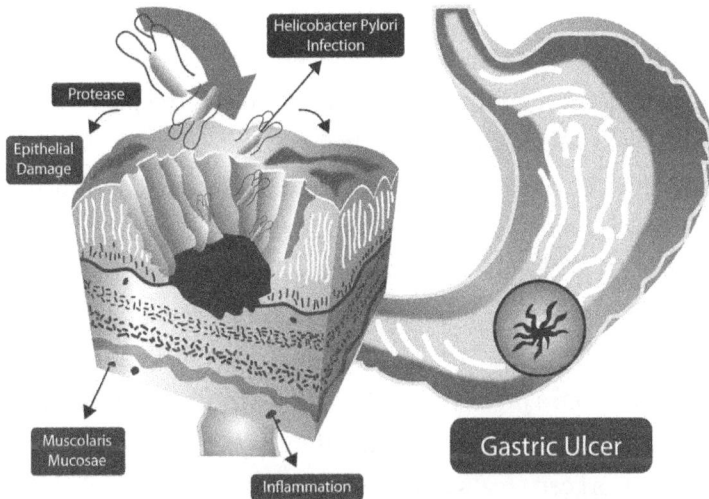

Imagine your H. pylori infection is like a canoe. You take antibiotics or antimicrobials to kill the infection, and the canoe (H. pylori) starts taking on water (medication or herbs). Your goal is to sink that canoe and kill the h. pylori. But the efflux pumps are like someone inside the canoe (inside the H. pylori) bailing the water back out into the ocean. So as long as the water (the antibiotics or herbal antimicrobials) can be bailed out as fast as it's coming in, the canoe can stay afloat—the H. pylori will survive. There are strategies you'll learn about in the chapter "The Infection Connection" that can be utilized to kill H. pylori better by knocking out or slowing down these efflux pumps.

H. pylori's Effect on the Gut

In the 1980s, Dr. Barry Marshall discovered that H. pylori was the primary driver of ulcers, and for his efforts he won a Nobel prize.[13] Before this, it was believed that ulcers were formed due to stress and too much stomach acid.

In reality, H. pylori produces an enzyme called *urease* that decreases the amount of stomach acid (raises the pH). Urease takes the protein, urea, that's being digested in the stomach, and then breaks it down into ammonia and carbon dioxide (CO_2). Ammonia has a high pH between 11 and 12. Ammonia's higher pH will lower the overall acidity in the stomach. The measurement of pH is on a scale of 1 to 14: 1 to 6 is acidic, 7 is neutral (water), and 8 to 14 is alkaline. Small changes matter as a change from a pH of 3 to a pH of 4 drops the acidity by a factor of ten times; the pH scale is logarithmic.

H. pylori can create inflammation in the gut, and inflammation can lead to gut permeability (leaky gut).

What Is a Leaky Gut?

The intestinal lining contains layers of cells connected by tight junctions. The intestinal lining is supposed to allow only the appropriate nutrients to pass through and into the bloodstream.

When the tight junctions become inflamed due to gluten, infections, or other irritating foods or toxins, they can open, and these same foods and infectious debris can slip through and enter the bloodstream. This is known as leaky gut, or gastrointestinal permeability as it is commonly referred to by the scientific community.[14] This is a gray area in conventional medicine and isn't a diagnosis taught in medical school, even though there are thousands of studies supporting it.

The bloodstream carries these toxins throughout your body, where they are absorbed in a variety of locations, creating inflammation. As offending foods continue to flood into the body, the leaky-gut cycle continues, keeping your body in a constant state of inflammation.

A leaky gut can create an immune response known as *molecular mimicry*. The surface proteins on gluten, for example, can look very similar to those of the thyroid and can cause a case of mistaken identity, or molecular mimicry, to occur. (This is true for other body tissues as well—dairy can look like the pancreas, for example.)

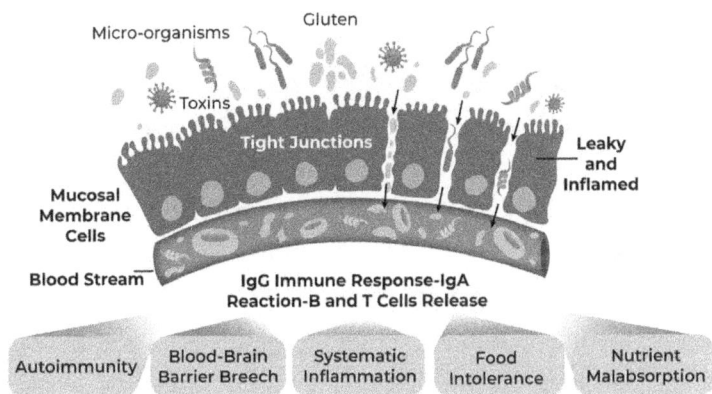

Micro-organisms · Gluten · Toxins · Tight Junctions · Leaky and Inflamed · Mucosal Membrane Cells · Blood Stream · IgG Immune Response-IgA Reaction-B and T Cells Release · Autoimmunity · Blood-Brain Barrier Breech · Systematic Inflammation · Food Intolerance · Nutrient Malabsorption

The immune system starts making antibodies for the thyroid because it can't tell the difference, and then the thyroid is under attack. Infection and a leaky gut are two of the prime mechanisms that exacerbate the breakdown of the thyroid.

Leaky gut can present itself in a variety of ways and can lead to chronic conditions. Some people may have irritable bowel syndrome (IBS), Crohn's disease, or other pathological conditions. Others may have skin issues, bloating, gas, or gastroesophageal reflux disease (GERD). Still others may fall somewhere in the middle.

When you have healthy gut function, your gut works like the oil filter in your car. When infections and undigested food particles slip through and enter the bloodstream, they are carried to the liver, the body's detoxification system, and that puts additional stress on the liver (we'll discuss this more in "The Liver Connection," a chapter later in the book).

When the tight junctions in your intestines become more permeable, it is like having oil in your car's engine without the oil filter. If your engine is missing its oil filter, the oil can thicken, become very gelatinous, and actually cause the engine to seize. In the gut, when cells get sticky due to inflammation, your ability to excrete fecal debris and toxins can slow down. So not only are toxins passing into your bloodstream and putting extra stress on the liver, but now your intestines are moving slower, which increases your chances of reabsorbing toxins in your stool.

Beneficial good bacteria (probiotics) in the gut are important for optimal immune and thyroid health. Good bacteria eat poop and poop out nutrition (excrete nutrients), while bad bacteria eat nutrition and poop out poop. In other words, good bacteria eat the bad stuff and produce good stuff, while bad bacteria eat the good stuff and produce bad stuff.

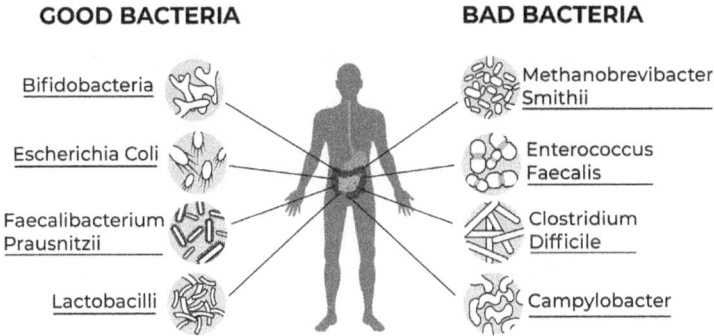

GOOD BACTERIA

Bifidobacteria

Escherichia Coli

Faecalibacterium Prausnitzii

Lactobacilli

BAD BACTERIA

Methanobrevibacter Smithii

Enterococcus Faecalis

Clostridium Difficile

Campylobacter

Common Gut Infections

It's not just bacteria that causes gut inflammation. Parasites, viruses, and yeasts are found in the gut as well. A few common infections, which will be discussed more in the infection chapter, are found when dealing with leaky gut. Thyroid issues follow these infections. A list of those infections include these:

- **H. pylori:** This bacterium is common in greater than 50 percent of the population and can drive autoimmunity contributing to Hashimoto's. It is linked to other autoimmune conditions and is transmitted through saliva or fecal contamination.[15]

- **Borrelia burgdorferi (Lyme disease):** This bacterium looks similar to the thyroid, so it can exacerbate autoimmunity and trigger diseases, such as Parkinson's and ALS. The deer tick is most commonly responsible for transmitting Lyme disease, which can be an acute or chronic infection.[16]

- **Yersinia enterocolitica**: This bacterial infection can trigger thyroid conditions and autoimmunity. It is transmitted through contaminated food and water.[17]

- **Candida**: This fungal infection disrupts digestion, throws off good–bad gut bacteria balance, and can create constipation. It is transmitted through direct contact and can be spread by contact with contaminated objects. Excess carbohydrate, refined sugar, and antibiotic use can drive candida overgrowth.[18]

- **Epstein-Barr virus (mono, the kissing disease)**: This virus causes an imbalance in the immune system and is present in 80 to 90 percent of the population. It's connected to many autoimmune conditions, including Hashimoto's and multiple sclerosis. It is transmitted through saliva.[19]

Healing a Leaky Gut

There are six strategies I like to follow when helping patients heal their leaky gut. I call it the *6R strategy*. There's a very specific order in which these strategies must be followed:

1. **Remove** hyperallergenic foods
2. **Replace** enzymes, acids, and bile salts
3. **Repair** the body with healing nutrients and adrenal support
4. **Remove** infections
5. **Reinoculate** with probiotics and prebiotics
6. **Retest** to ensure the infection has cleared

Let's explore each of these more in depth.

Remove Hyperallergenic Foods

The first step is to remove all irritating foods that can contribute to a leaky gut. This would include foods that are nutrient-poor, high in inflammation, and elevated in toxins. Physical, chemical, and emotional stressors can lead to inflammation, and inflammation tends to cause our bodies to break down faster. Irritating, hyperallergenic foods introduce physical and chemical stressors to the body.

Stressors cause the *immunoglobulin A* (IgA) in the mucosal barrier in the gut lining to break down. When this happens, sinus infections, gut issues, irritation, fungal infections, or even urinary tract infections may appear. Removing irritating foods can help remove this stress from the gut.[20]

The foods to remove vary from individual to individual. Commonly irritating foods include, but are not limited to, the following:

- Grains
- Sugar
- Dairy
- GMO foods
- Processed foods
- Non organic foods

If there is an autoimmune issue as well, you may need to add a rotation component to the diet and also eliminate foods that include the following:

- Nuts
- Seeds
- Tomatoes

- Potatoes
- Eggplants
- Peppers

Again, there's not a one-size-fits-all plan here. Each person has to find his or her offending food and eliminate it.

Since 70 to 80 percent of the immune system is located in the gut, via the GALT (gastric associated lymphoid tissue) in the stomach or the MALT (mucosal associated lymphoid tissue) in the small intestine, removing allergenic foods is particularly important for keeping the gut healthy and taking stress off the immune system.[21]

Replace Enzymes, Acids, and Bile Salts

When the body is overstimulated by the sympathetic nervous system (SNS)—when your foot hits the gas pedal—it's in a fight-or-flight state. As you get more stressed, your blood rushes toward the extremities so you can fight or flee.

As blood leaves your digestive system, you are less able to produce the enzymes, hydrochloric acid (HCl), and bile salts needed for proper digestion. This makes the environment more susceptible to dysbiosis, small intestinal bacterial overgrowth (SIBO), and chronic infections.

Your parasympathetic nervous system (PNS) is in the rest-and-digest state—your foot is on the brake. The PNS actually brings the blood inward toward the gut, and this allows for proper enzyme, HCl, and bile salt production. This shows us that getting your body back under the control of the PNS is important.

Repair with Healing Nutrients, Adrenal and Hormone Support

There are specific healing nutrients that will help repair the gut. When there is significant inflammation in the gut along with chronic gut infections, it is always smart to add extra healing support to calm down the intestinal tract and immune system first. Some of my favorite gut nutrients are L-glutamine, slippery elm, marshmallow root extract, aloe vera, zinc, and licorice, which are soothing and will assist with reducing inflammation and promoting healing in the gut. The enterocytes, the cells that make up your gut barrier, love L-glutamine and glycine, which are key nutrients in bone broth and can be very healing for the gut lining as well.

Having healthy adrenal glands is also very important for healing the gut. The adrenals produce cortisol, which helps neutralize inflammation and maintain a healthy gut lining. If you have too much cortisol due to inflammation in the body, that elevated cortisol can weaken your gut lining. If your cortisol function is too low, it will be harder to generate energy and repair your gut lining.

Having an appropriate stress response through healthy adrenal function is important. Cortisol is produced to help deal with inflammation, so if there is inflammation in the gut, cortisol can also put out that flame before it grows into a five-alarm fire. The more cortisol is stimulated, the more it can decrease your sex hormone output. These sex hormones not only help with reproduction, but they also help with healthy aging. As your healthy aging hormones drop—including DHEAs, testosterone, estrogen, and progesterone—we may notice less muscle mass, less skin elasticity, and a slower recovery from physical activity.

Remove Infections

Removing infections is imperative, and this step is often missed in traditional medicine. Infections can drive a leaky gut, keeping us in a stressed-out state, which keeps the SNS activated, preventing digestion.

Blood work and a comprehensive stool analysis are two tests that should be done to determine if there is an infection and what exactly the infection is (SIBO, dysbiosis, bacteria, parasites, etc.).

When most people find out they have a gut infection, they make the mistake of saying, "Oh, my! I have to get rid of this infection." Then they take every antibiotic or herbal medicine under the sun to knock it out, and they end up feeling worse. We live in a society that has a track record of overprescribing antibiotics, which is what has created this trigger-happy reaction, understandably.

There is a reason why removing infections is near the bottom of my step-by-step list of strategies: it can actually be stressful to your detoxification system, lymphatic system, and immune system to remove an infection too soon.

In some people, the hormonal system (adrenals, thyroid, and male or female hormones) must be addressed first to decrease the risk of side effects and other issues. It's important to do steps 1 through 3 first, as they strengthen the body's constitution, which makes the biotoxins from the infections less stressful and more manageable in step 4 (remove).

Reinoculate with Probiotics

Imagine you have a backyard garden full of weeds. It's difficult to plant new seeds in a weedy garden. There's not enough room for those seeds to grow. You're going to have to pull out the weeds and prepare the soil before you can plant your new seeds.

In these first four strategies, the weeds (bad stuff) are removed, and the soil (your gut) is prepared. Now reseeding (reinoculating) can occur, and the good bacteria are put back in. These beneficial bacteria don't live forever; they tend to hang around for a month or so before they pass through your intestinal tract. That's why getting exposure to good, fermented food and/or supplemental probiotics is very important for lasting, healthy gut function long-term.

Many people with SIBO develop symptoms when probiotics are added first, like bloating, gas, and brain fog, to name a few. These issues occur when seeds are planted in a garden full of weeds. Get the first four steps in check first, and then introduce probiotics into a gut with a fertile, receptive environment. Some patients who are very probiotic sensitive do better with low-histamine and spore-based probiotics. These probiotics tend to be less reactive for sensitive patients and still have positive effects on the gut microbiome.

Retest to Ensure the Infection Has Cleared

Make sure you retest for the original infection. Some people need second and third treatment rounds to clear the infection completely while other people even end up with a new infection from a microbe that burrowed deeper into the gut lining and finally made its way to the surface after the previous infection was cleared.

> **Pro tip:** If you have chronic gut issues, it is especially important to get your partner tested and treated, as it can be very easy to pass infections back and forth. Some infections, like H. pylori, can even be spread via saliva, which makes them extremely easy to pass on to a family member when drinks and eating utensils are shared.

Testing for Gut Issues

There are a number of tests that can be used to look for proper gut function, infections, and problems, such as leaky gut or gut permeability. These include blood tests, comprehensive stool tests, SIBO breath tests, and transit-time tests.

Blood Tests

Basic blood tests can indirectly assess protein absorption. These tests include the typical complete blood count (CBC) and comprehensive metabolic profile (CMP). These tests will also report on levels of creatinine, albumin, globulin, and blood urea nitrogen (BUN). They will even assess some of your immune markers, like neutrophils, lymphocytes, eosinophils, basophils, and monocytes, which give clues on how well your immune cells are responding.

I have a reference handout on blood testing ("Blood Test Review") that you are welcome to download. You can find it in the resources section at the end of the book.

Comprehensive Stool Test

H. pylori			
Helicobacter pylori	2.6 E4	High	<7.0 E3
Virulence Factor, cagA	Negative		Neg
Virulence Factor, vacA	Positive		Neg

Parasites by PCR	Quantitation	Units	Assay Range	Results
Blastocystis hominis	47	MFI	10–5000	Negative
Entamoeba histolytica	688	MFI	10–5000	Positive
Giardia spp.	94	MFI	10–5000	Negative
Trichomonas spp.	30	MFI	10–5000	Negative

Fungi/Yeast		
Candida albicans	<dl	<5.0 E3
Candida spp.	Negative	Neg
Geotricum spp.	Mod	Neg
Microsporidia spp.	Negative	Neg
Trichosporon spp.	Negative	Neg

Private patient lab

I recommend running a DNA stool test. DNA stool tests can amplify infections that may get missed when looking at them under a microscope, like older stool antigen tests would. The advantage of these tests is that the lab test requires only one sample and a very small amount of the infectious debris to detect it.

These tests can also give us a window into immune markers like immunoglobulin A levels (IgA), calprotectin, eosinophil activation protein (gut inflammation markers), and steatocrit (fat digestion marker), to name a few. To access my preferred lab tests, see the resources section at the end of the book. Lab technology is constantly evolving, so my recommendations may change over time.

SIBO Breath Test

In a SIBO (small intestinal bacterial overgrowth) breath test, a sugar solution (lactulose) is given to the patient. The test measures the time it takes for the lactulose to move through the intestinal tract and the gases produced by the potentially bad bacteria when consumed.

For instance, you would blow into a tube to measure your baseline. You would then take a lactulose sugar solution (a large sugar molecule that you can't digest, so the only thing that's able to break it down is the gut bacteria). You blow into the tube every twenty minutes for three hours (at 0 minutes, then 20, 40, 60, 80, 100, 120, 140, 160, and 180), and you get readings of the methane and hydrogen gases at these various times. At the 120-minute mark, the lactulose should be able to reach the end of the small intestine, where it starts to enter the large intestine (colon). If there is an overgrowth in the small intestine where bad bacteria migrate up from the colon, the bacteria will start to eat the lactulose solution, causing the production of methane or hydrogen gas, depending on the bacteria. An increase in methane and hydrogen is normal after the 120-minute mark as the lactulose has already reached the large intestine (colon).

These gases are nothing more than an indirect marker that bad bacteria are present. The gases aren't just naturally there at these levels. They are there because of the overgrowth of bad bacteria from the large intestine up to the small intestine. If there's an abundance of methane, it can potentially slow down motility, leading to constipation. If there's an elevation of hydrogen gas, it can typically accelerate motility, causing diarrhea. And if both gases are present, symptoms may alternate between constipation and diarrhea.

You can access the SIBO breath test I prefer through the link in the resources section at the back of the book.

Urinary Organic Acids

Urinary organic acids are another way to assess dysbiotic bacterial overgrowth. There's no way to know for sure the exact location of the dysbiotic bacteria, so we can't officially say SIBO is present, which is very location-specific to where the bad bacteria are. This test still gives another noninvasive indicator that general dysbiosis may be present. This test can also be helpful in discovering Clostridium difficile metabolites, candida, colonized mold, and fungal overgrowth metabolites, which can be easily missed on a stool test.

Urinary organic acids can also help look at markers outside of the gut, including mitochondrial nutrients, neurotransmitters, methylation, and detoxification pathways. In future

Small Intestinal Bacterial Overgrowth (SIBO) 3 Hour Lactulose

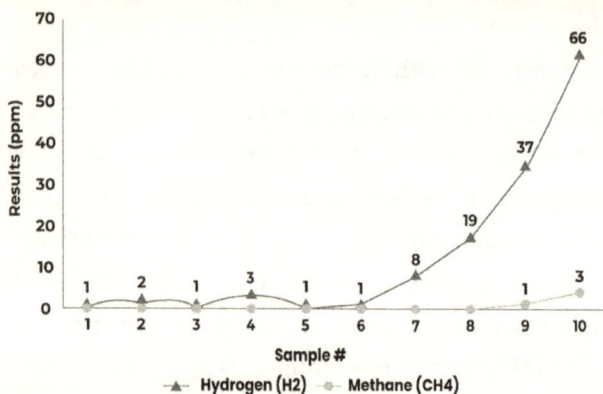

Hydrogen (H2)   Methane (CH4)

Collection Time	ppm H2	ppm CH4	SUM H2 AND CH4	CO2*
Baseline	1	0	1	OK
20 min	2	0	2	OK
40 min	1	0	1	OK
60 min	3	0	3	OK
80 min	1	0	1	OK
100 min	1	0	1	OK
120 min**	8	0	8	OK
140 min	19	0	19	OK
160 min	37	1	38	OK
180 min	66	3	69	OK

· Samples are corrected for Carbon Dioxide (CO_2) concentration to account for variants in collection. Invalid samples are categorized as Quantity Not Sufficient (QNS).

**120 minutes is the typical time at which the biomarker travels from the small intestine to the colon. However, slow transit times will result in SIBO marker during the last hour.

Summary of Results

Trace Gas Markers:	Result (ppm):	Guideline:	Interpretation:
Baseline Hydrogen (H2)	1	Normal:<=20 ppm	Normal
Greatest Hydrogen (H2) rise over lowest previous value in first 120 minutes	7	Normal:<=20 ppm	Normal
Greatest Methane (H2) rise over lowest previous value first 120 minutes	0	Normal:<=12 ppm	Normal
Greatest rise in the combined sum of Hydrogen (H2) and Methane (CH4) over lowest previous sum in first 120 minutes	7	Normal:<=15 ppm	Normal
Peak Methane (CH4) at any point in the test	3	Normal:<=3 ppm	Normal

Private patient lab

chapters, we will come back to the topic of organic acid testing and how it can be helpful in assessing and supporting thyroid function.

COMPOUNDS OF BACTERIAL OR YEAST/FUNGAL ORIGIN

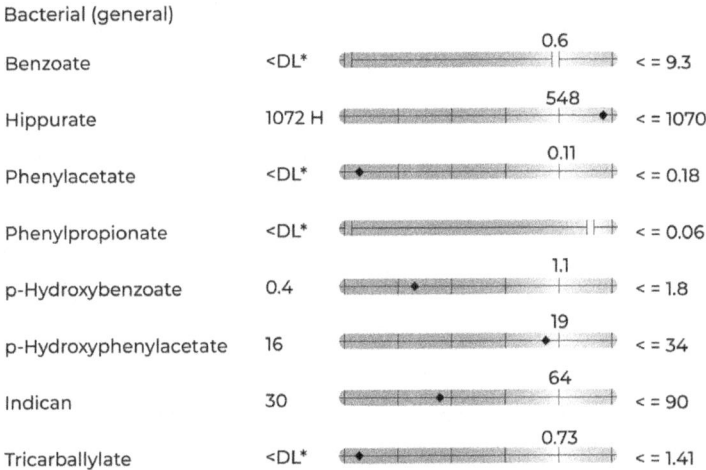

Bacterial (general)

Benzoate	<DL*	0.6	< = 9.3
Hippurate	1072 H	548	< = 1070
Phenylacetate	<DL*	0.11	< = 0.18
Phenylpropionate	<DL*		< = 0.06
p-Hydroxybenzoate	0.4	1.1	< = 1.8
p-Hydroxyphenylacetate	16	19	< = 34
Indican	30	64	< = 90
Tricarballylate	<DL*	0.73	< = 1.41

Private patient lab

Transit Time Test

Transit time tests measure the time it takes from food entering your mouth to being eliminated in a bowel movement. The test can typically be done by consuming some beets or charcoal. You set the time as you eat. Ideally, within eighteen to twenty-four hours, you want to produce a bowel movement that's black if you consumed charcoal or red if beets.

If it takes less than eighteen hours, it could be a sign of malabsorption and indicates that your bowels are moving too fast, like in the case of diarrhea. If it takes over twenty-four hours and you're not passing at least twelve inches of stool per day, you may be reabsorbing the toxins from the stool, potentially creating a problem known as *autointoxication*, where you are adding to your toxic load. A lot of what's in your stool are toxins bacteria and fiber. The body needs to move that material out to maintain optimal health.

KEY POINTS

1. Healthy stomach acid lowers the pH in the stomach. When you have healthy stomach acid, it starts a cascade supporting optimal digestion.

2. Thyroid hormone is instrumental in helping to create peristalsis, and one major symptom in hypothyroidism (low thyroid hormone) is constipation.

3. As you continue to feed your body offending foods, the leaky-gut cycle continues, keeping your body in a constant state of inflammation and malnutrition.

4. Healthy gut bacteria are the key because good bacteria eat poop and poop nutrition, while bad bacteria eat nutrition and poop poop.

5. Follow this step-by-step 6R approach to healing the gut: remove hyperallergenic foods; replace

enzymes, acids, and bile salts; repair with healing nutrients and adrenal support; remove infections; reinoculate with probiotics; and retest to ensure the infection has cleared.

Resources

Thyroid Reboot Foundations Bundle (www.justinhealth. com/foundations) Here are several recommended thyroid-supporting supplements mentioned in the book in easy-to-access bundles.

Digestive Support (www.justinhealth.com/digestive) These are some digestive-supporting supplements that I recommend to my patients, ranging from digestive acids to enzymes, and bile support to gut-healing nutrients.

Health Tracker (www.justinhealth.com/health-tracker) Here, you can efficiently manage and track your previous lab work. Additionally, there is an API feature that allows you to connect to your health insurance portal and upload PDFs of old lab tests. These documents will be automatically transcribed and uploaded to your portal, including graphed lab values, which will make it easier for you to assess your lab trends.

Comprehensive Stool Test (www.justinhealth.com/stool-test) This is a genetic stool test that I recommend that uses sensitive PCR DNA technology that will detect bacteria including H. pylori, parasites, and fungal overgrowth.

This test also assesses gut inflammation, immune function, enzymes, and fat malabsorption.

SIBO Breath Test (www.justinhealth.com/breath-test) This is a lactulose breath test that will test for methane and hydrogen gas production to help assess small intestinal bacterial overgrowth.

Organic Acid Test (OAT) (www.justinhealth.com/organic-acid-test) This test looks at organic acids, giving us a window into the function of metabolic processes in the body like detoxification, mitochondrial function, nutritional deficiencies, gut bacteria, and fungal overgrowth.

Comprehensive Blood Test (www.justinhealth.com/comprehensive-blood-test) This is a comprehensive blood test that includes a CBC, metabolic panel, full thyroid panel, vitamin D panel, inflammation panel, and urinalysis.

Complete Thyroid Test (www.justinhealth.com/complete-thyroid-test) This is a comprehensive thyroid panel, including TSH, T4 free, T4 total, T3 free, T3 total, TPO ab, TG ab, and RT3.

Abridged Thyroid Test (www.justinhealth.com/abridged-thyroid-test) This is an abridged thyroid panel including TSH, T4 free, T3 free, TPO ab, and TG ab.

H. pylori Breath Test (www.justinhealth.com/h-pylori-breath-test) This is an H. pylori breath test to help detect H. pylori.

Micronutrient Test (www.justinhealth.com/micronutrient-test) This is a test that will look at blood and urine to assess micronutrient levels.

Iron Test (www.justinhealth.com/iron-test) This is a comprehensive iron test looking at ferritin, iron saturation, IBC, iron total, and reticulocyte count.

Notes

1   Selma P. Wiertsema et al., "The Interplay between the Gut Microbiome and the Immune System in the Context of Infectious Diseases throughout Life and the Role of Nutrition in Optimizing Treatment Strategies," *Nutrients* 13, no. 3 (2021): 886, https://doi.org/10.3390/nu13030886.

2   Marcel Mazur et al., "Autonomic Nervous System Activity in Constipation-Predominant Irritable Bowel Syndrome Patients," *Medical Science Monitor* 18, no. 8 (2012): CR493–99, https://doi.org/10.12659/msm.883269.

3   Yasuhiro Koga, "Microbiota in the Stomach and Application of Probiotics to Gastroduodenal Diseases," *World Journal of Gastroenterology* 28, no. 47 (2022): 6702–715, http://dx.doi.org/10.3748/wjg.v28.i47.6702.

4   Olga Yaylali et al., "Does Hypothyroidism Affect Gastrointestinal Motility?," *Gastroenterology Research and Practice* 2009 (March 7, 2010): 529802, https://doi.org/10.1155/2009/529802; and Mazur et al., "Autonomic Nervous System Activity."

5   Aryn B. Collins and Roman Pawlak, "Prevalence of Vitamin B-12 Deficiency among Patients with Thyroid Dysfunction," *Asia Pacific Journal of Clinical Nutrition* 25, no. 2 (2016): 221–26, https://www.airitilibrary.com/Common/Click_DOI?DOI=10.6133%2fapjcn.2016.25.2.22.

6   Abdul Jabbar et al., "Vitamin B12 Deficiency Common in Primary Hypothyroidism," *Journal of the Pakistan Medical Association* 58, no. 5 (May 2008): 258–61, https://pubmed.ncbi.nlm.nih.gov/18655403.

7   Michael B. Zimmermann and Josef Köhrle, "The Impact of Iron and Selenium Deficiencies on Iodine and Thyroid Metabolism: Biochemistry and Relevance to Public Health," *Thyroid* 12, no. 10 (July 9, 2004): 867–78, https://doi.org/10.1089/105072502761016494.

8   Jagmohan Hooda, Ajit Shah, and Li Zhang, "Heme, an Essential Nutrient from Dietary Proteins, Critically Impacts Diverse

Physiological and Pathological Processes," *Nutrients* 6, no. 3 (2014): 1080–102, https://doi.org/10.3390/nu6031080.

9   Masayoshi Yamaguchi, Toshiharu Yoshino, and Shoji Okada, "Effect of Zinc on the Acidity of Gastric Secretion in Rats," *Toxicology and Applied Pharmacology* 54, no. 3 (July 1980): 526–30, https://doi.org/10.1016/0041-008X(80)90180-5.

10   Afshin Shafaghi et al., "The Effect of Zinc Supplementation on the Symptoms of Gastroesophageal Reflux Disease; a Randomized Clinical Trial," *Middle East Journal of Digestive Diseases* 8, no. 4 (2016): 289–96, https://doi.org/10.15171/mejdd.2016.38.

11   Elizabeth A. Grice and Julia A. Segre, "The Human Microbiome: Our Second Genome," *Annual Review of Genomics and Human Genetics* 13 (September 2012): 151–70, https://doi.org/10.1146/annurev-genom-090711-163814.

12   Atin Sharma, Vivek Kumar Gupta, and Ranjana Pathania, "Efflux Pump Inhibitors for Bacterial Pathogens: From Bench to Bedside," *Indian Journal of Medical Research* 149, no. 2 (February 2019): 129–45, https://pubmed.ncbi.nlm.nih.gov/31219077.

13   Barry Marshall, "Helicobacter pylori--a Nobel Pursuit?," *Canadian Journal of Gastroenterology and Hepatology* 22 (2008): 459810, https://doi.org/10.1155/2008/459810.

14   David M. Brady, ""Autoimmune Disease: A Modern Epidemic? Molecular Mimicry, the Hygiene Hypothesis, Stealth Infections, and Other Examples of Disconnect between Medical Research and the Practice of Clinical Medicine,"" *Townsend Letter* 347 (June 2012): 45–50, https://www.diagnosticsolutionslab.com/sites/default/files/Autoimmune%20Disease-Modern%20Epidemic-Brady%20DM-Townsend%20Letter%202012%20%282017_06_09%20 15_12_54%20UTC%29.pdf.

15   Konstantinos X. Papamichael et al., "*Helicobacter pylori* Infection and Endocrine Disorders: Is There a Link?," *World Journal of Gastroenterology* 15, no. 22 (June 14, 2009): 2701–707, http://dx.doi.org/10.3748/wjg.15.2701.

16   Nyembezi Dhliwayo et al., "Lyme Disease: An Autoimmunity-Based 'Destructive Thyroiditis' or Just Another 'Non-Thyroidal Illness'?," *Journal of the Endocrine Society* 5, suppl. 1 (April–May 2021): A940–41, https://doi.org/10.1210/jendso/bvab048.1922.

17 Moein Zangiabadian et al., "Associations of Yersinia Enterocolitica Infection with Autoimmune Thyroid Diseases: A Systematic Review and Meta-Analysis," *Endocrine, Metabolic, & Immune Disorders: Drug Targets* 21, no. 4 (June 21, 2020): 682–87, http://dx.doi.org/10.2174/1871530320666200621180515.

18 Piotr Bargiel et al., "Microbiome Metabolites and Thyroid Dysfunction," *Journal of Clinical Medicine* 10, no. 16 (2021): 3609, https://doi.org/10.3390/jcm10163609.

19 Michael P. Pender, "The Essential Role of Epstein-Barr Virus in the Pathogenesis of Multiple Sclerosis," *Neuroscientist* 17, no. 4 (2011): 351–67, https://doi.org/10.1177/1073858410381531.

20 Bernadeta Pietrzak et al., "Secretory IgA in Intestinal Mucosal Secretions as an Adaptive Barrier against Microbial Cells," *International Journal of Molecular Sciences* 21, no. 23 (2020): 9254, https://doi.org/10.3390/ijms21239254.

21 Wiertsema et al., "The Interplay between the Gut Microbiome and the Immune System."

4

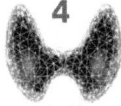

The Adrenal Connection

THE ADRENALS AND THYROID FUNCTION TOGETHER, but they also can dysfunction together. When one of them is not happy, it can drag the other one down. This is why adrenal balance is imperative to optimal thyroid health.

The adrenals are your stress-handling glands. They help the body manage and deal with stress. One of the primary stress hormones the adrenal glands create is *cortisol*. Cortisol is a *glucocorticosteroid*. *Gluco* pertains to blood glucose and the body's ability to generate energy; *corticosteroid* pertains to your body's ability to manage inflammation. There are natural corticosteroids for pain and inflammation; for example, a cortisone injection may be used for a painful shoulder or knee. Your body produces cortisol, a sister substance to cortisone.

Cortisol is needed for energy and to help with inflammation. When stressed, most people don't manage it properly, whether physically, chemically, or emotionally. Your adrenals are called to the rescue. Their job is to either create energy or deal with putting out the fire. That's one part of the adrenals. The other part of the adrenals acts as the backup battery or backup generator for sex hormone production.

The adrenals also produce a hormone called *DHEA sulfate* (DHEAs), which is a precursor to many of the sex hormones, such as estrogen, progesterone, and testosterone. Sex hormones are important not only for reproduction but also for helping us heal our bodies and minds on a daily basis. These hormones also play a significant role in muscle building and neurological health. If you're stressed, without rebuilding hormones you won't be able to rebuild muscle and brain neurons that are important to help you think.

The thyroid is like the resting tone of a car while in neutral. If the RPM or the engine is running too slowly, the car can stall. If the car is running too fast or too hot, it can redline and burn out. The adrenals are akin to shifting the car's gear from first to second to help generate energy and deal with stress. Also, downshifting is akin to being able to relax, repair, and adapt to stress.

It's an intimate balance between a healthy engine tone and the engine's ability to speed up and slow down. If your own metabolic engines are missing this capacity, symptoms like fatigue, anxiety, poor mood, poor sleep, weight gain, PMS, hot flashes, and digestive problems can occur.

Adrenal Dysfunction and Fatigue

Common symptoms seen in adrenal dysfunction and fatigue include depression, mood issues, digestive issues, sleep problems, joint pain, headaches, excessive allergies, the inability to lose weight, the inability to deal with stress, and low libido. Because a significant amount of sex hormones are produced by the adrenals, PMS or an exacerbation of menopausal symptoms like hot flashes, dry skin, and hair loss often show up in females when the adrenals are out of balance.

Most people with adrenal fatigue don't get help from their conventional medicine doctor or their endocrinologist, who refer to adrenal fatigue as Addison's disease or adrenal failure. I prefer the term *adrenal dysfunction*, as it is more descriptive of the functional high and low cortisol swings that I tend to see clinically in practice. Some patients may have lower cortisol in the morning but higher cortisol at night. With adrenal dysfunction, there is usually a combination of an adrenal rhythm problem (the time when cortisol is produced in the morning, noon, afternoon, and night) as well as how much cortisol is produced overall throughout the day. Even sex hormone precursors like DHEAs can be depleted as well. Adrenal problems tend to point to something deeper upstream.

Conventional medicine conducts tests that look at end-stage, or pathological, adrenal cortisol levels, like the extreme lows of adrenal cortisol in Addison's disease or the extreme highs of adrenal cortisol in Cushing's. These conditions typically involve a brain or adrenal tumor, like in Cushing's, or an autoimmune condition, like in Addison's. This is much different than what we are talking about here with functional adrenal dysfunction. If you want some additional information on the topic, feel free to watch my video at the end of the chapter. In your car you have a light on your dashboard that signifies when something with the car is not right. A conventional medical doctor, when it pertains to the adrenal for instance, sees the light on as being equivalent to adrenal disease, and the light off means you are healthy with no disease. In summary, light on = disease, light off = healthy.

The problem with this analogy is that health is not binary (on or off); it exists on a continuum, just like a dimmer switch controlling that same dashboard light. You could have the light turned on 90 percent, but if it's not 100 percent on, it won't get picked up under a conventional assessment as being a problem. You've probably heard of patients who are told, "It's all in your head" or "You're just getting older." These are people who instinctively know something is wrong, yet they still fall through the cracks of the conventional medical system.

Functional medicine looks at the origin of the stress—the lifestyle stressors, the nutritional imbalances, and so on—that are leading up to the gland not working properly or dysfunctioning.

As a functional medicine doctor, I'm not treating disease; I'm not a medical doctor. I am addressing the underlying physical, chemical, and emotional stressors that cause dysfunction before a disease can manifest.

The Different Layers of the Adrenal Glands

Here is a quick tip to help you remember the layers of the adrenal glands that I learned in doctoral school. Salt, sugar, and sex—the deeper you go, the better it gets. I am confident now you will never forget how the adrenals work.

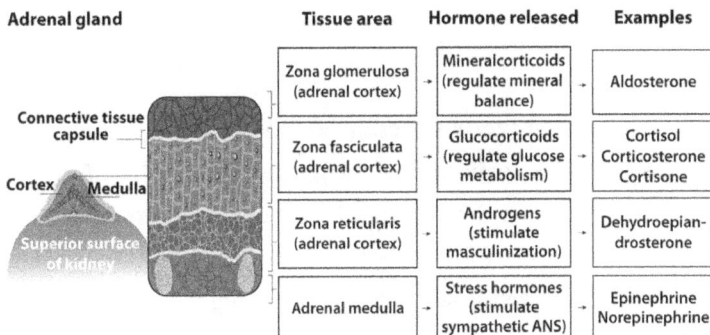

Adrenal gland	Tissue area	Hormone released	Examples
Zona glomerulosa (adrenal cortex)	Mineralcorticoids (regulate mineral balance)	Aldosterone
Zona fasciculata (adrenal cortex)	Glucocorticoids (regulate glucose metabolism)	Cortisol Corticosterone Cortisone
Zona reticularis (adrenal cortex)	Androgens (stimulate masculinization)	Dehydroepian-drosterone
Adrenal medulla	Stress hormones (stimulate sympathetic ANS)	Epinephrine Norepinephrine

- **Outer layer (zona glomerulosa):** This layer pertains to the mineralocorticoids aldosterone which help you hold onto minerals like sodium and potassium. Minerals are very important for cellular physiology like with your sodium/potassium pumps. These minerals are also important so your nervous system can function properly and so we can maintain healthy blood pressure levels. When there is adrenal stress and inflammation, it is common to dump minerals like potassium which can increase dizziness, heart issues, and muscle cramping. Insulin resistance can make this worse by the way.

- **Middle layer (zona fasciculata):** This layer pertains to your glucocorticoids (or, less commonly, glucocorticosteroids) like cortisol. Cortisol has a dual function; it can help manage and mobilize blood sugar, and it can also act as an anti-inflammatory when there is excessive inflammation. Cortisol when chronically used to fight inflammation can break down muscle, tissue, ligaments, and bone.

- **Inner layer (zona reticularis)**: This layer produces a sex hormone precursor known as DHEA (dehydroepiandrosterone). DHEA can help provide building blocks for testosterone in men, and it can also help provide sex hormone building blocks like estrogen in women. DHEA levels from the adrenal are very important for menopausal women, because when the ovaries stop producing sex hormones, the adrenals are relied on more to fill in the gap. Women who enter menopause with weaker adrenal function tend to have more menopausal symptoms like hot flashes, mood issues, hair loss, and lower libido.

- **The innermost layer (adrenal medulla)**: This layer produces adrenaline which kicks the sympathetic nervous system into gear. Adrenaline is a fast-acting stress hormone and opens the floodgates for cortisol as well. Adrenaline and cortisol work together; when cortisol is high, adrenaline tends to be high too. Adrenaline is also known as a *catecholamine* and *epinephrine*. (I know—lots of words that mean the same thing can be confusing sometimes.)

Adrenal Stress and Healing

In addition to cortisol, the adrenals produce many other hormones, and one of the major hormones is *pregnenolone*, which is considered the mother of all steroid hormones. Pregnenolone is the building block for over twenty different adrenal hormones in the hormonal cascade. This pregnenolone can become depleted over time because it is being used to make stress hormones like cortisol. Over time, this makes it harder for the body to manage and handle stress. Maybe you've seen this in your own life when different stressors begin to pile up, whether it's a poor diet, work stress, or family stress. You may find your tolerance to new stress drops to zero.

Your brain is hardwired to make calculations and prioritize which stressors it should be allocating resources to. Putting on muscle, recovering from and healing aches and pains, and having high amounts of energy may all get put on the back burner until these immediate stressors are addressed. Healing and repair are for tomorrow, but stress, which has to be dealt with now, is the body's priority.

Healing and repair always benefit you the next day; you never feel the benefits in the moment. Typically, healing and repair in the moment make you tired. It feels like you're sore. This occurs because your body is in a parasympathetic recovery state. It's not until two or three days later that you feel the full rejuvenating effects of the repair process. For many people, it can take weeks before they notice improvement. The longer these immediate stressors go unaddressed, the longer your body procrastinates healing. Like a middle-school kid studying for a test, it tends to get put off until the last minute. Many people do the same; they wait until the symptoms are so intense and real before they decide it's time to do something about it.

Your body is hardwired to deal with inflammation and stress in the moment. How? With building blocks.

Imagine your body has building blocks sitting there, ready to get to work on the inflammation and stress. These building blocks are called pregnenolone. Pregnenolone is only one step downstream from cholesterol, which is why healthy fats and proteins, especially from healthy, organic animal products, are vital. Without those building blocks providing the proper amount of pregnenolone, optimal performance will be harder to achieve.

If inflammation is chronic (ongoing), the body switches tracks from the regenerative healing process and focuses on inflammation and stress. It has to prioritize these building blocks toward reducing inflammation because they are a higher priority at the moment. Survival is always the body's number one priority; without it, we wouldn't exist today.

One of the first things we deal with when looking at adrenal issues is how to quench the inflammation and stress of the moment so your adrenals can help with repair and recovery tomorrow. *You have to intervene and stop the inflammation and stress before any healthy healing and recovery can happen.*

In the image below, you can see the stress hormone pathway, which leads to cortisol and its weaker metabolite, cortisone. The female hormone pathway leads primarily to estrogen and progesterone (higher in women). The pathway that leads to testosterone and androgens is higher in men. This should give you a good idea of how the adrenal hormone cascade flows downstream to make all of your different hormone building blocks.

STEROID HORMONE SYNTHESIS PATHWAYS

Adrenal glands

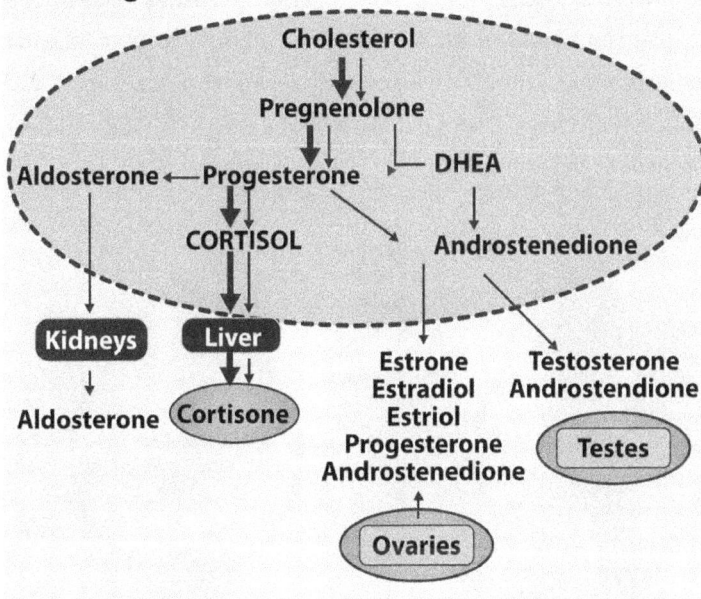

Why Is Cortisol So Important?

Healthy adrenal function means healthy cortisol levels and cortisol rhythm throughout the day. Due to the influence of light and darkness on your natural circadian rhythm, cortisol is naturally higher in the morning. This means that cortisol is higher in the morning to provide energy to get out of bed and lower at night before bed so you can wind down and fall asleep.

Cortisol production is also needed for the thyroid to convert inactive thyroid hormone T4 to active thyroid hormone T3. If cortisol levels are too high, this will decrease T4-T3 conversion and potentially cause the pituitary to increase TSH production (your brain hormone). Your brain hormone, which talks to your thyroid, increases because your brain thinks you are in a stressed-out state. It does its best to yell downstream, similar to a parent talking to their kids while they are making a lot of noise; instinctively, they raise their voice so their kids will hear them over the commotion.

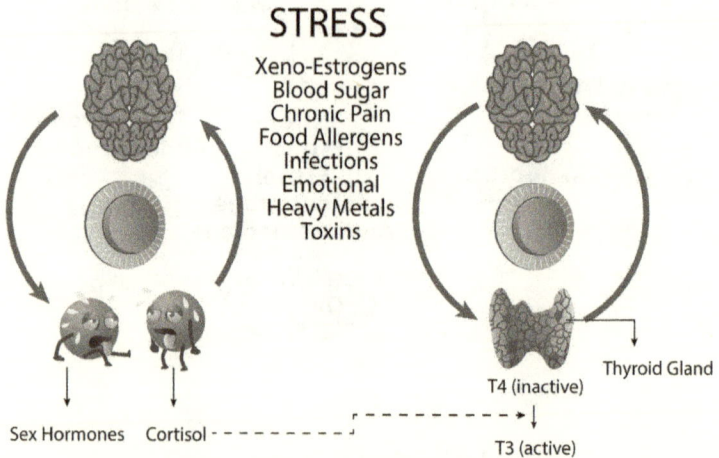

STRESS
Xeno-Estrogens
Blood Sugar
Chronic Pain
Food Allergens
Infections
Emotional
Heavy Metals
Toxins

Thyroid Gland

T4 (inactive)

Sex Hormones   Cortisol

T3 (active)

Over time, if cortisol levels continue to drop because chronic stress and inflammation won't stop, the upstream pituitary finally just says, "All right, forget it. I'm just going to take a nap." And it, too, starts to drop production. Optimal thyroid hormone conversion can't happen without the proper amount of cortisol.

Cortisol and the HPA Axis

A lot of people who have chronic stress have an upstream hypothalamus and pituitary that are sleeping because they're just tired of the stress. It's like a thermostat. The thermostat is set at 70 degrees, your stress capacity. If it gets too hot, it goes to 75 degrees, and the air conditioner kicks on and brings down the temperature; if it gets too cold, the heat kicks on and the temperature comes back up.

If the thermostat stops working—if your ability to manage stress (our hypothalamus and pituitary) stops working optimally—the heat and the air conditioning won't turn on when they should. They stop doing their job. Now you wouldn't say that the heater or the air conditioner is broken—what you would say is that the command center and the thermostat (the hypothalamus, pituitary, and brain) aren't working optimally. They are stressed out.

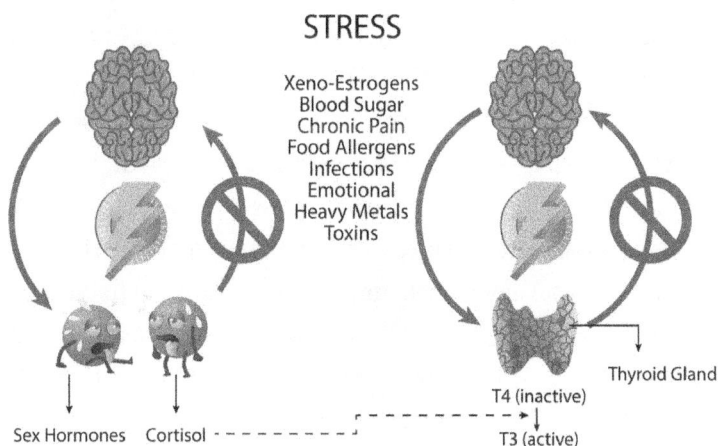

STRESS

Xeno-Estrogens
Blood Sugar
Chronic Pain
Food Allergens
Infections
Emotional
Heavy Metals
Toxins

Thyroid Gland

T4 (inactive)

Sex Hormones   Cortisol

T3 (active)

Many people actually have HPA—hypothalamus, pituitary, and adrenal—axis dysfunction. When this happens, it's the brain's communication with the adrenals that is dysfunctional, not the adrenals themselves. The HPA axis is not working because the body is saying, "You know what? I'm too tired. I'm tired of talking to these screaming kids. I'm taking a nap." When the HPA axis is not functioning properly, the adrenals can't properly produce the cortisol required for thyroid hormone conversion. On the flip side, cortisol levels may be so high that we can't tamp down the cortisol levels, thus decreasing thyroid hormone conversion through excess cortisol.

Cortisol's Effect on Other Body Functions

Do you recall the thyroid hormonal cascade from Chapter 1? Twenty percent of thyroid hormone conversion happens in the thyroid, and the other 80 percent happens peripherally, or elsewhere in the body. One of those peripheral locations is the liver, where detoxification is controlled. We need healthy cortisol levels for detoxification to help deal with the potential inflammation from the phase 1 detox metabolites. You also need healthy cortisol levels for proper gut function, because if your gut doesn't have the ability to deal with stress and inflammation due to food intolerances, indigestion, or a food allergen, then the gut may not be able to heal and recover properly.

Your cortisol levels can impact your immunoglobulin A (IgA) levels, the mucosal membrane antibody barrier that lines the gut. If cortisol levels are too high, you'll burn through your IgA barrier. If cortisol levels are too low, the production of IgA can become impaired. IgA provides a barrier of protection against invaders, whether they're bacteria, parasites, viruses, or fungi.

Remember, if your gut is not working optimally, dysbiosis is a possibility, which is an imbalance of the bad bacteria in the gut. With an increase in the ratio of bad gut bacteria and not enough beneficial bacteria, there could be a decrease in intestinal sulfatase enzymes. The intestinal sulfatase is produced by beneficial bacteria and is responsible for converting T3S (*T3 sulfate*) and T3AC (*T3 acetic acid*) into active T3 thyroid hormone.[1]

Factors Affecting the Adrenals

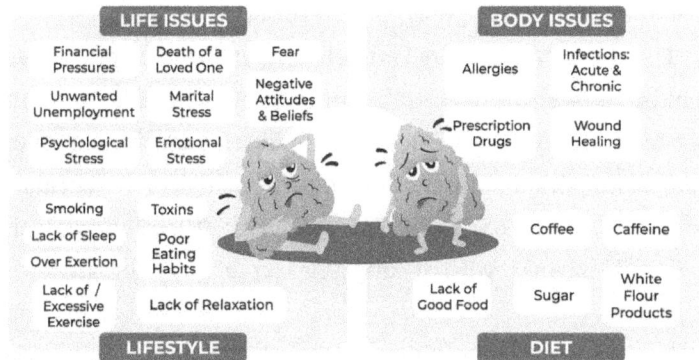

LIFE ISSUES				BODY ISSUES	
Financial Pressures	Death of a Loved One	Fear		Allergies	Infections: Acute & Chronic
Unwanted Unemployment	Marital Stress	Negative Attitudes & Beliefs			
				Prescription Drugs	Wound Healing
Psychological Stress	Emotional Stress				
Smoking	Toxins				
Lack of Sleep	Poor Eating Habits			Coffee	Caffeine
Over Exertion					
Lack of / Excessive Exercise	Lack of Relaxation			Lack of Good Food	Sugar	White Flour Products
LIFESTYLE				DIET	

Without healthy cortisol levels, your body has a decreased ability to adapt to stress. This can increase the chance of more thyroid hormone being converted to reverse T3 (inactive thyroid hormone), the metabolic blanks in the gun we discussed in Chapter 1.

If cortisol is elevated, typically that's a sign of an acute physical, chemical, or emotional stressor: exposure to a parasite, stress at school, a fight with a spouse, poor food choices, or even overexercise. Most people can adapt to these stressors and come back to a level of stability or homeostasis.

A significant number of people go from one stressor to the next, and over time, these stressors begin to accumulate and compound. It's common to have at least some awareness of the emotional stress in life, like work, financial, or family stress; it tends to be the chemical stress that falls under people's radar as it is not able to be easily perceived. It is exceedingly difficult to pinpoint these types of stress without the help of a well-trained functional medicine practitioner to help you navigate the situation. The blog post "Adrenal Fatigue vs. Failure" in the resources section is a great place to start.

The chemical stressors I am referring to could be pesticides, molds, xenoestrogens, or other unnatural chemicals found in our food supply. It could be that your blood sugar is on a roller coaster ride throughout the day, going from high to low because your meals aren't balanced. This stress can cause low stomach acid and enzyme levels, making it harder for you to break down your food.

Not getting enough quality sleep could be another root cause of stress. Impaired sleep makes it harder to repair and recover and can increase your body's accelerated breakdown. People go from one stressor to another, and acute short-term stress starts to turn into chronic long-term stress. Chronic stress can increase inflammation in your body, impair your immune system, and make you more susceptible to infections.

The Adrenals and Blood Sugar

One of the biggest stressors on the thyroid and adrenals is blood sugar. The adrenal hormone cortisol is a glucocorticoid (*gluco-* pertains to its ability to impact blood sugar and energy and reduce inflammation). If blood sugar levels are out of balance from skipping meals, eating too much refined sugar, or eating too many inflammatory foods like grain, pasteurized dairy products, and foods that are too high in sugar, you can end up on a blood sugar roller coaster called *reactive hypoglycemia*.

When too much sugar hits the bloodstream in a short time frame, the pancreas squirts out a whole bunch of insulin to help bring that blood sugar into the cell. The faster your blood sugar goes up, the faster you produce insulin, and the more insulin you produce. Insulin brings sugar into the cell—that's the goal. If you bring blood sugar into the cell too fast, your blood sugar level can bottom out.

Many people have a hard time wrapping their heads around the fact that eating sugar can actually cause low blood sugar. They think sugar will make their blood sugar go up. Yes, this does happen—in the first thirty minutes to maybe an hour. But what's the long-term effect? The long-term effect is that the surge in blood sugar bottoms out, and you will actually create a low blood sugar environment.

Low blood sugar is a stress signal to your body and can stimulate your adrenal glands to produce more adrenaline (catecholamines or epinephrine), which is another stress hormone your adrenals make outside of cortisol. Adrenaline works very fast and can cause you to feel anxious and jittery. After adrenaline is produced, it will cause your cortisol levels to increase a few minutes later, bringing your blood sugar back into balance. When this high adrenaline and insulin starts to become a pattern, it can damage your metabolism and hurt your thyroid.

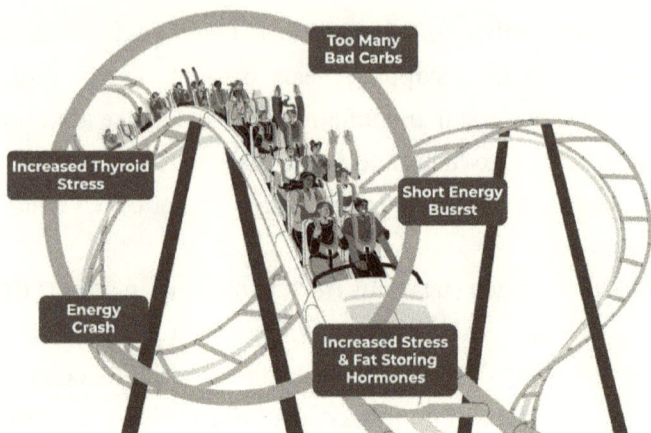

Many people who have chronic fatigue and chronic health issues are literally living their whole lives on this blood sugar roller coaster. They go from one meal to the next on this high-to-low blood sugar dip.

Your conventional doctor may tell you to have some candy on hand to bring your blood sugar up. This is not the answer. All it does is bring your blood sugar back up temporarily, and a few hours later you crash even harder. Then it's more difficult to break the blood sugar roller coaster cycle.

The more your adrenal glands are called to the rescue, the more dysregulated your adrenals become. Cortisol, which is produced from your adrenals, has an anti-inflammatory effect on the body when produced, while at the same time it can mobilize glucose and increase your blood sugar levels. Too much cortisol can create chronically high blood sugar levels and initiate the breakdown of lean tissue and muscle in your body. Essentially, your adrenals are a double-edged sword; the less you use them at the extremes, the better off you are.

The more the adrenals are stimulated due to blood sugar imbalances and inflammation, the more stress the brain is under to help the body adapt (HPA axis—hypothalamus, pituitary, adrenal feedback loop).[2] But that is not all. Your thyroid also becomes stressed. Blood sugar is an important aspect of healthy thyroid hormone conversion.

Type 2 diabetics, by definition, have chronically elevated blood sugar levels due to insulin resistance. These same diabetics also show a strong association with lower thyroid hormone levels, most notably low T3 levels. We talked about cortisol being intimately involved in T4 to T3 thyroid conversion and activation, but high levels of insulin, as seen in type 2 diabetes, can impair thyroid conversion too.[3]

If you stay on the blood sugar roller coaster too long, you will chronically shift from high to low blood sugar levels throughout the day. Over time, your cells will become resistant to the high levels of insulin, thus causing chronically high blood sugar levels. This downward spiral continues to negatively impact your thyroid, as your cortisol and insulin imbalances only get worse over time if the problem isn't addressed.

Managing the Stress: Conservation versus Abundance

High levels of adrenaline and stress hormones will affect thyroid hormone conversion. Why? When under stress, you need fuel for your body to perform optimally, and you don't want to produce stress hormones that will compete for the same fuel your thyroid needs.

Think of thyroid hormone as high-octane gasoline. Thyroid hormone increases your metabolism and the temperature of your body, allowing your body to generate more energy by burning more fuel. The healthier your metabolism is, the more your body can tap into ketones and body fat for fuel. The more stress you put on your body, the more your thyroid begins to downregulate your metabolism with the goal of conserving the fuel it's burning so it has more resources to handle stress in the future.

Think about how you might go about managing the finances of your household. If you have an abundance of money coming into your bank account, you can go out to dinner, take a vacation, and buy some new furniture. You can be a little bit more extravagant with the things you purchase. But what if you lose your job or have some extra expenses because some unexpected bills are due? Then you have to really manage your expenses more prudently and maybe develop an emergency fund to avoid this situation in the future.

It's the same thing with your body. When you are stressed, you have to be very careful about how many extra stress hormones your body creates and how much energy your body will need to conserve. During stress, the body should be in a state of conservation rather than a state of spending, just like you would conserve and save your money when finances are strapped.

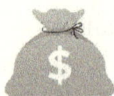

| Finances Tight | | Finances Abundant |
| Conserve Money | | OK to spend |

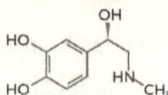

Adrenaline

| Body Stressed | | Body Healthy |
| Conserve Energy | | OK to Use Energy |

Managing stress physically, chemically, and emotionally to create an ideal hormonal environment within the body is important. It's critical to figure out what key stressors are active and make sure you are taking steps to address them. It's also important to have optimal hormone levels to help support muscle mass, healthy brain function, optimal digestion, and mitochondria. This type of environment allows your body to adapt to the stress coming its way. This provides an anabolic environment where your body has a surplus of optimal health reserves (an emergency fund) and has the capacity to weather the down times if they come.

The more you can signal your body to be in a state of abundance, the better you feel physically, chemically, and emotionally; the better your sex hormones function; and the better your libido, energy, focus, mood, and brain function will be. Basically, the healthier you are, the better you can roll with the punches and adapt to the stress life throws at you.

When Lions Attack: The Microstress Effect

When lions attack, there is a short life-or-death stress period for their prey. If they survive, a minute later they are back to eating again, grazing calmly in the fields. Most of the stress humans deal with is chronic stress (physical, chemical, and emotional) that lingers throughout the day, weeks, months, and so on.

The process of detoxification requires healthy levels of cortisol. If cortisol is too high, detoxification can be impaired. High cortisol levels equal stress. When you're stressed, your brain and body treat it as though you are running from a tiger, so to speak, so why would detoxifying or even something as essential as digestion be a priority?

We're not running from tigers today, but let's face it, when sitting in traffic for an hour while people cut us off, we're responding as if under stress, like a mini tiger is after us.

Another mini tiger could be the boss yelling at you, skipping breakfast in the morning, getting into an argument with a spouse, or even missing an hour or two of sleep. The list could also include exposure to a food allergen like gluten or having impaired digestion due to a gut infection like H. pylori.

Realistically, there are many mini tigers that arise all day long. They aren't real tigers, so you don't feel a sense of being eaten alive, but these mini tigers add up, and they can become even worse over time than that one big tiger. With a big tiger, you either evade it and live, or it eats you. Either way, the situational stress is quickly gone—you don't have to worry about it anymore.

On the other hand, the microstress builds up and has an impact on your stress-handling glands that is worse than a large tiger chasing you. It makes you susceptible to chronic diseases, including thyroid and adrenal imbalances.

Controlling the Effects of Microstress

There are many ways to control the effects of microstress while keeping the adrenal glands functioning appropriately. These methods go back to the three stressors in our Triple-S Approach covered in Chapter 1:

1. **Manage emotional stress:** Nurturing your relationships with work colleagues, family, and friends is a major way to do this. Use prayer, meditation, talk therapy, journaling, or other psychological techniques like EMDR

(eye movement desensitization and reprocessing) or EFT (emotional freedom technique) to process emotional stress and create a state of gratitude in your life.

2. **Manage chemical stress**: Blood sugar dysregulation is one of the biggest stressors on the hormonal system. Managing blood sugar by eating every four to five hours and choosing the right fuel mixture—protein, fat, and carbohydrates—to stabilize your blood sugar is the best way to do this. Eating foods that are anti-inflammatory, nutrient dense, and low in toxins through organic whole foods is another way to manage chemical stress exposure.

3. **Manage physical stress**: Getting to bed before 10:30 p.m. and sleeping at least seven to eight hours seems simple, and it's one of the best ways to manage physical stress. Choosing exercise that allows you to feel energized after your workout is completed is important too. Make sure you can emotionally recover from your exercise to the point where you could comfortably repeat the movement again if you needed to. Make sure you don't feel like you were hit by a bus the next day. You should not feel excessively sore the day after your workout unless you are doing a new exercise you don't typically do.

Tests for the Adrenal Glands

The *cortisol rhythm test* is a saliva or urine test that looks at the free fractions of cortisol produced throughout the day. The total fraction of cortisol can also be assessed, typically through urine or blood only. Cortisol samples are taken at specific times throughout the day, the first being around breakfast (between 6:00 and 8:00 a.m.), at lunch (between 12:00 and 1:00 p.m.), in the afternoon (between 4:00 and 5:00 p.m.), and at bedtime (between 10:00 p.m. and midnight). This test shows us how cortisol fluctuates throughout the day and can give us insight into your HPA axis function. Cortisol levels are on a circadian rhythm triggered by light-and-dark cycles as discussed in Chapter 2.

Functional Adrenal Stress Profile

Parameter	Result	Reference Range	Units
Cortisol - Morning (6 - 8AM)	12.9*	13.0 - 24 0	nM/L
Cortisol - Noon (12 - 1PM)	7.5	5.0 - 8.0	nM/L
Cortisol - Afternoon (4 - 5PM)	3.6*	4.0 - 70	nM/L
Cortisol - Nighttime (10PM - 12AM)	3.1*	1.0 - 30	nM/L
Cortisol Sum	27.1	23.0 - 42 0	nM/L
DHEA-S Average	15.30*	2.00 - 10.00	ng/mL
Cortisol/DHEA-S Ratio	1.8*	5.0 - 6.0	Ratio

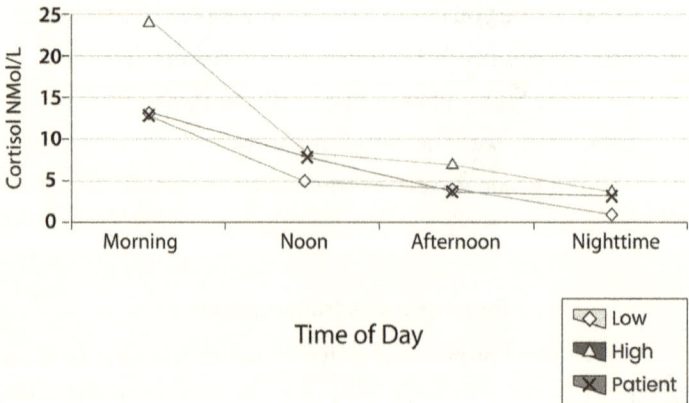

Low
High
Patient

Remember, sunlight triggers cortisol production in the morning. When cortisol rises, you generate energy to get out of bed, and then cortisol gently tapers down throughout the day, allowing you to wind down and produce melatonin to help you fall asleep.

To evaluate adrenal function, the rhythm and the total amount of cortisol produced throughout the day are important to look at. Why is adrenal rhythm important? When we start to see the adrenals lose that normal circadian rhythm in regard to a high-to-low cortisol taper throughout the day, it's one of the first signs of HPA axis dysfunction (think back to the thermostat analogy). When cortisol starts to deviate from its expected rhythm, symptoms like fatigue, depression, anxiety, and insomnia can follow. Higher cortisol levels are associated with anxiety, irritability, and insomnia. Lower cortisol levels can be associated with fatigue, depression, and mood issues. It is also possible to be somewhere in between, with a combination of high and low cortisol production throughout the day at different times, even with normal cortisol levels for the daily output. Cortisol rhythm matters: it impacts your mood and energy.

Assessing cortisol levels, whether free or total, independent of the time of day can be helpful in assessing adrenal function and gland strength. Lower levels of cortisol production, usually in the bottom 25 percent of the reference range, can be a reliable sign of adrenal dysfunction; higher productions of cortisol in the top 25 percent of the reference range may provide an indication that the adrenals are under acute stress.

Different labs have different reference ranges, so assessing where you fall within the functional range as a percentage or standard deviation is more important than referencing actual lab ranges.

The original theories of adrenal fatigue were developed by Hungarian endocrinologist Dr. Hans Selye and are called the *general adaptation syndrome.*[4] Selye used the stress curve as shown below to explain how stress affects hormones and the immune system over time. Chronic stress over time creates a maladaptive physiological response, partly contributing to adrenal fatigue and a hypo-cortisol environment or depleted cortisol levels.

Over time, we have come to understand that the adrenals aren't fatigued or depleted like Selye thought, like in Addison's disease or adrenal failure. Instead, the lower levels of cortisol reflect HPA axis dysfunction or a disruption in the communication feedback loops from the brain to the adrenal glands. I see many patients with low levels of free cortisol, while at the same time the total levels of cortisol are still quite adequate. Clinically, this is important because, as we deal with stress, we aren't just supporting healthy adrenal function but also healthy communication throughout the hormonal system, including the thyroid. When it comes to hormones, everything functions and dysfunctions together.

FYI: Free cortisol is not bound to a protein and represents 2 to 5 percent of all cortisol in your body. Total cortisol represents 2 to 5 percent of free cortisol and the other 95 to 98 percent of protein-bound cortisol as well.

Stress Curve Phases (General Adaptation Syndrome)

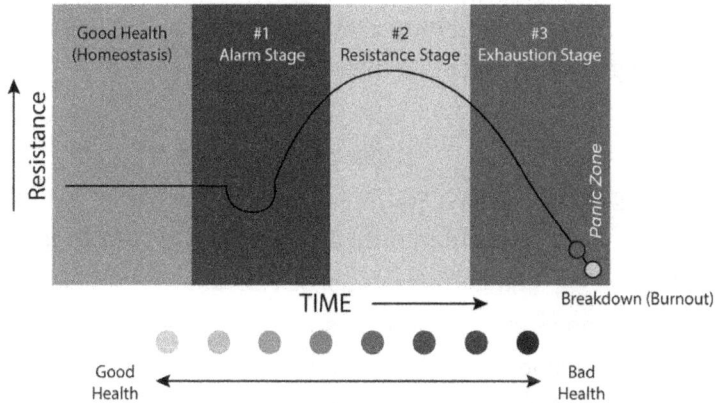

Stages of Adrenal Dysfunction

Stage 1

Free and total cortisol levels begin to elevate. You may also see an increase in DHEA (the sex hormone precursor made by the adrenal glands), which is a response to the high levels of cortisol. DHEAs can help lower high levels of cortisol. When cortisol is elevated, there is usually some type of acute stress response. It's important to look at all underlying physical, chemical, and emotional stressors when supporting the adrenals with supplementation to ensure the root cause is still being addressed. Typical symptoms may include anxiety, increased belly fat, brain fog, insomnia, and a hard time relaxing.

Stage 2

Cortisol levels stay around midrange, but you may start to see cortisol rhythm aberrations, whether high or low, throughout the day. These rhythm issues indicate that there may be HPA dysfunction—the brain is not communicating properly to the adrenals. Typical symptoms may include depression, anxiety, brain fog, fatigue, and other digestive symptoms.

Stage 2/3

This stage is like Stage 2, with some notable exceptions, including a decrease in sex hormones. We may start to see a drop in either free or total cortisol levels. Sex hormones like DHEAs start to drop as chronic adrenal stress increases; healing and repair become less of a priority, and stress and inflammation become a greater priority. Typical symptoms may include depression, anxiety, brain fog, fatigue, PMS, and other digestive symptoms.

Stage 3

Cortisol rhythms start to track lower, flatter, and, in some cases, even reverse. With a reverse cortisol rhythm, cortisol starts out extremely low to start the day and may even run higher at night, making it harder to wind down at night while still feeling tired during the day. Free and total cortisol levels run low, and sex hormones like DHEA run low as well. If we are testing sex hormones like progesterone, estrogen, and testosterone, these may also run low. The adrenals at this point are very depleted due to chronic stress and inflammation. Typical symptoms may include depression, anxiety, brain fog, fatigue, an inability to recover after workouts, a harder time building muscle and losing weight, PMS, and menopausal symptoms. As you progress through the adrenal stages, symptoms tend to increase and spread to other body systems, like digestion.

It is important to remember that the adrenals never dysfunction at random. There is always some root physical, chemical, or emotional stressor at play, whether obvious or not. It's the job of a skilled functional medicine practitioner to help uncover what those stressors may be while at the same time supporting your adrenals and hormonal systems, providing the optimal healing environment.

Functional medicine support
Pregnenolone, DHEA, licorice, vitamin C with bioflavonoids, B_5, B complex, phosphorylated serine, adaptogens like holy basil, ashwagandha, rhodiola, eleuthero, maca, magnesium, GABA, multivitamin support, and L-theanine, to name a few, are all possible options.

All functional medicine support and dosage should be individualized for the patient. Other tests may be run to fine-tune the supplement recommendations above or beyond just an adrenal or hormone panel. Not all supplements on the recommendation list should be used. The list is designed to show you the different types of support that could be used. Specific doses are not given due to the uniqueness of each patient.

Hormone Testing

What is always exciting to me is that there's a constant evolution in the world of functional medicine. There is newer testing technology that becomes available that assesses adrenals and hormones in a much deeper way that allows us to view free cortisol as well as total cortisol in the same sample, unlike salivary cortisol testing, which only allowed us to view free fractions

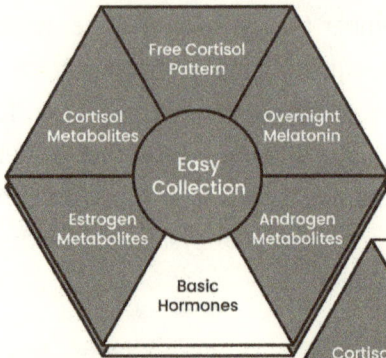

Blood Testing

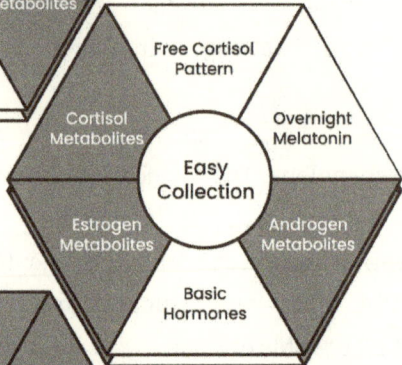

Easy Collection
- Free Cortisol Pattern
- Overnight Melatonin
- Androgen Metabolites
- Basic Hormones
- Estrogen Metabolites
- Cortisol Metabolites

Saliva Testing

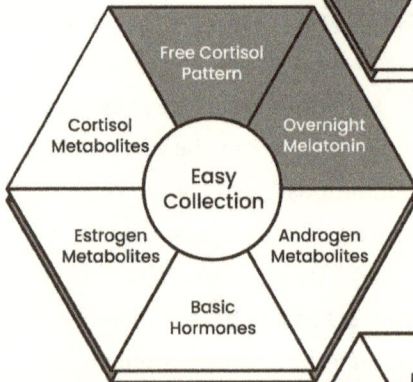

Easy Collection
- Free Cortisol Pattern
- Overnight Melatonin
- Androgen Metabolites
- Basic Hormones
- Estrogen Metabolites
- Cortisol Metabolites

24-Hour Urine Testing

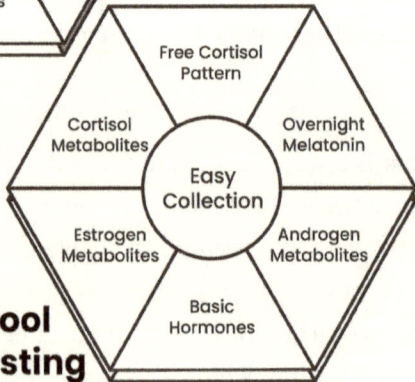

Easy Collection
- Free Cortisol Pattern
- Overnight Melatonin
- Androgen Metabolites
- Basic Hormones
- Estrogen Metabolites
- Cortisol Metabolites

Free End Tool Hormone Testing

Easy Collection
- Free Cortisol Pattern
- Overnight Melatonin
- Androgen Metabolites
- Basic Hormones
- Estrogen Metabolites
- Cortisol Metabolites

of hormones. We can also look at hormone detoxification as well as other complete sex hormones. The previous graphic depicts this difference among the testing methods, which we will address later in the chapter. To access my preferred lab tests, see the resources section at the end of the book. Lab technology is constantly evolving, so my recommendations may change over time.

It's helpful to see if free cortisol and total cortisol levels match up (both fall in a similar area of the reference range). Sometimes we may see high free cortisol and low total cortisol, which may signify low thyroid or iron levels. Other times we may see the reverse: low free cortisol and high total cortisol, which may signify a more significant HPA axis dysfunction issue.

Most of the adrenal dysfunction cases I see are more complicated and may involve multiple body systems like the thyroid, digestion, and detoxification. To get optimal success with patients, you need to start with a solid foundation, including diet and lifestyle, as you address other major stressors (physical, chemical, and emotional) while working through the body's systems (hormones, gut, and detox). The biggest mistake I see with patients that come to me from other doctors is that they work through more complicated protocols for infection killing or detoxification without a solid foundation first. Just like when building a house, the taller and bigger the home, the more solid the foundation needs to be.

There are more antiquated schools of thought that address adrenal fatigue through the concept of "the pregnenolone steal," where building blocks of the adrenal hormones are shunted to make stress hormones like cortisol. This results in fewer building blocks for sex hormones and an inability to repair them. Low-hormone symptoms like PMS, low libido, fatigue, insomnia, and mood disorders are also common.

Adrenal Hormones

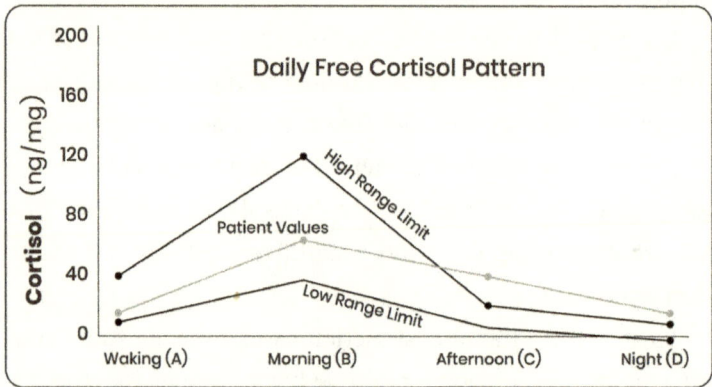

Free cortisol best reflects tissue levels.
Metabolized cortisol best reflects total cortisol production.

Total DHEA Production

Age	Range
20-40	800-2500
40-60	530-1550
>60	400-1350

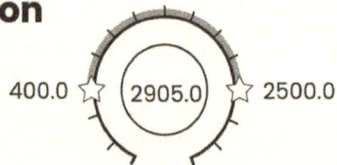

400.0 ☆ 2905.0 ☆ 2500.0

Total DHEA Production
(DHEAS + Etiocholanolone + Androsterone)

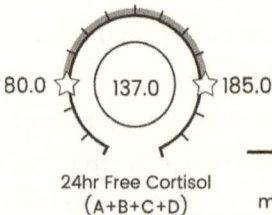

80.0 ☆ 137.0 ☆ 185.0

24hr Free Cortisol
(A+B+C+D)

→ cortisol metabolism

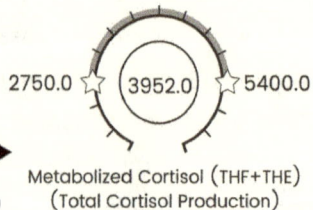

2750.0 ☆ 3952.0 ☆ 5400.0

Metabolized Cortisol (THF+THE)
(Total Cortisol Production)

As we have addressed earlier in the chapter, the result of adrenal dysfunction is more of a chronic communication disruption from the brain to the adrenals (HPA-axis dysfunction). This is why it's so important to use nutrients and supplement support that nourishes the adrenal glands as well as supports healthy communication with the brain, adrenals, and thyroid.

Conventional Medicine's Flawed Approach to Testing

Conventional medical doctors will typically assess adrenal issues by running a *serum cortisol test* from the blood rather than a free-fraction cortisol test from urine or saliva. The problem with this is that 2 to 5 percent of hormone fractions are free. Serum represents 95 to 98 percent of the protein-bound hormone. When they're running a serum test, they're looking at glandular output with the goal of detecting a disease in the organ—usually an autoimmune condition or a tumor that affects the adrenals or pituitary, like in Addison's or Cushing's disease.

There is another problem with the serum cortisol test. It involves a blood draw and is usually only taken once a day in the morning. Most people say they get nervous and stressed out when they are in a doctor's office, especially when getting a needle jabbed into their arm. Take a guess at what this stress does to their stress hormone level while they are there. It can increase your stress hormones and may give you a higher-than-normal reading on your cortisol test.

Now take the situation of someone who may have had lower stress hormones to start with. Along comes this needle stress that may give you an artificial boost to your stress hormone levels, throwing off your hormone results. Because this is a one-time-only blood test, not a saliva or urine test done multiple times to assess cortisol rhythm, we lose the ability to get a window into the HPA axis function. Completing multiple test samples throughout the day, using a non-stressful collection method, provides cleaner and more useful results. This helps your functional medicine doctor understand what is happening in your body and create a better plan to fix it.

Conventional doctors will usually also do an *ACTH stimulation test* to assess adrenal disease. In this test, a drug or a compound (Cosyntropin) is given to the patient to stimulate their adrenals to see if they can make more cortisol. It's like whipping a tired horse; you would expect the horse to giddy up and move with that kind of stimulation, and if it doesn't, you can assume you're dealing with a pair of tired and diseased adrenal glands.

Most people I see are not in a state of adrenal failure. They are typically experiencing a functional imbalance, usually in between a state of optimal health and disease. So essentially, these people are stuck in no man's land, and they don't get the help they need because their test results look normal. Basically, they are told their illness is all in their heads, and stimulants or even antidepressants may be recommended to control the symptoms. The problem with this approach is that the underlying causes of why they feel the way they do are ignored and almost always continue to get worse over time.

Cold Therapy—Thyroid and Adrenal Function

Utilizing cold plunges, which involve immersing yourself in water temperatures ranging from 40 to 50 degrees Fahrenheit, can significantly benefit the adrenals, thyroid, and nervous system.[5] The initial contact with cold water stimulates the adrenal glands to produce adrenaline, cortisol, and dopamine. This response can make you feel alert and energized, increasing the body's metabolic rate.

As your body adjusts to the cold, the parasympathetic nervous system becomes activated. This system drives blood inward as a protective response to keep your organs warm, promoting relaxation and calmness. It also lowers blood pressure and heart rate while boosting metabolism as your body works to raise its temperature to counteract the cold. This process can enhance adrenal function, thyroid hormone production, and conversion.

The great advantage of cold plunges—or even cold showers— is that they require minimal time to yield benefits. You can perform cold plunges in just three minutes, a few times a week. I will provide a link to my recommended cold plunge setup in the reference section at the end of this chapter and book. As an alternative, consider trying cold showers: switch to the coldest setting for ten to sixty seconds at the end of your hot shower each morning. Give it a week, and you're likely to find it invigorating. I've been taking cold showers for over a decade and have recently transitioned to cold plunges over the past year.

KEY POINTS

1. Consume the proper balance of proteins, fats, and carbohydrates to help manage metabolism and blood sugar. The more you create a blood sugar roller coaster, the more stress you put on your adrenals.

2. Go to bed before 10:30 p.m., and sleep at least eight hours. This helps support a healthy circadian rhythm for the adrenals.

3. Choose foods that are anti-inflammatory, nutrient dense, and low in toxins, utilizing our thyroid reboot diet. This will help your adrenal glands to heal.

4. Participate in exercise that is physically and mentally restorative rather than exercise that is depleting. Answer in the affirmative to the questions below:
    a. Make sure your exercise causes you to feel the same or more energized than when you started.
    b. Make sure you can emotionally repeat the exercise after completion. Once you have caught your breath, you should feel like you could complete it again.
    c. Make sure you are not overly tired or sore the next day after your workout. Newer movements that could cause more soreness are the exception.

5. Have your adrenals tested so you can be placed on the right adrenal program that improves your adrenal and thyroid health. Remember, the adrenals and thyroid function and dysfunction together.

Resources

Thyroid Reboot Foundations Bundle (www.justinhealth. com/foundations) Here are several recommended thyroid-supporting supplements mentioned in the book in easy-to-access bundles.

Urinary Adrenal Test (www.justinhealth.com/urine-adrenal-test) This is a comprehensive adrenal test that looks at free and total cortisol levels, cortisol rhythm throughout the day, and DHEA levels.

Urinary Complete Hormone Test (www.justinhealth.com/ urine-complete-hormone-test) This is a comprehensive adrenal test that looks at free and total cortisol levels, cortisol rhythm throughout the day, and DHEA levels. It also looks at progesterone, estrone, estradiol, estriol, testosterone, androgen metabolites, estrogen detox pathways, and six organic acid tests.

Urine Sex Hormone Test (www.justinhealth.com/urine-sex-hormone-test) This test will look at progesterone, estrone, estradiol, estriol, testosterone, androgen metabolites, and estrogen detox pathways.

Adrenal Support (www.justinhealth.com/adrenal) These are some of the adrenal nutrients that I recommend to my patients, ranging from botanicals to nutrients, and glandulars to bioidentical hormones.

Adrenal Fatigue versus Failure (www.justinhealth.com/ adrenal-fatigue-vs-adrenal-failure) This blog post compares the misconceptions between adrenal fatigue or dysfunction and adrenal failure.

Cold Plunge (www.justinhealth.com/cold-plunge) Has many metabolic benefits to increase metabolism and supporting a health parasympathetic nervous system response.

Notes

1   Jovana Knezevic et al., "Thyroid-Gut-Axis: How Does the Microbiota Influence Thyroid Function?," *Nutrients* 12, no. 6 (2020): 1769, https://doi.org/10.3390/nu12061769; and Rildo Guilherme de Oliveira Gomes, "Major Influences of the Gut Microbiota on Thyroid Metabolism: A Concise Systematic Review," *International Journal of Nutrology* 16, no 2 (March 2023), https://doi.org/10.54448/ijn23203.

2   Catherine J. Dunlavey, "Introduction to the Hypothalamic-Pituitary-Adrenal Axis: Healthy and Dysregulated Stress Responses, Developmental Stress and Neurodegeneration," *Journal of Undergraduate Neuroscience Education* 16, no. 2 (Spring 2018): R59–60, https://www.ncbi.nlm.nih.gov/pmc/articles/PMC6057754.

3   Chih-Yuan Wang et al., "Low Total and Free Triiodothyronine Levels Are Associated with Insulin Resistance in Non-Diabetic Individuals," *Scientific Reports* 8 (2018): 10685, https://doi.org/10.1038/s41598-018-29087-1.

4   Mark Jackson, "Evaluating the Role of Hans Selye in the Modern History of Stress," in *Stress, Shock, and Adaptation in the Twentieth Century*, D. Cantor and E. Ramsden, eds. (Rochester, NY: University of Rochester Press, 2014), https://www.ncbi.nlm.nih.gov/books/NBK349158.

5   Zhi Zhang et al., ""TRH Neurons and Thyroid Hormone Coordinate the Hypothalamic Response to Cold,"" *European Thyroid Journal* 7, no. 6 (2018): 279–88, https://doi.org/10.1159/000493976.

5

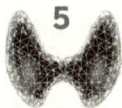

The Gluten Connection

DURING THE YEARS LEADING INTO WORLD WAR II, Dutch physician Dr. Willem Karel Dicke was working in hospital wards with children that were extremely sick. Dr. Dicke noticed that these patients got better during the wartime rations. Part of the plan for rations included no wheat, barley, or rye.

Once the war ended and the rations ended, the kids got sick again. Dr. Dicke eventually made the connection that these foods—wheat, barley, and rye—had

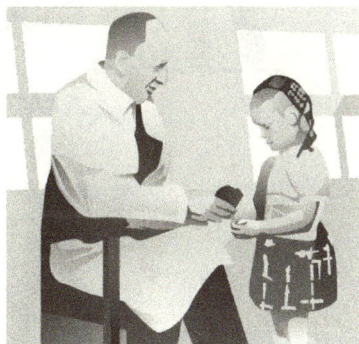

some type of inflammatory reaction that was keeping these kids from getting better.[1]

Flash forward seventy-five years. We now know that gluten is a strong agitator, or strong stimulator, for autoimmunity. Autoimmunity is the most common mechanism by which the thyroid gland gets attacked and inflamed. If this attack isn't quelled, the thyroid will lose the ability to function optimally over time, and symptoms like fatigue, hair loss, weight gain, digestive issues, and poor sleep, to name a few, can occur.

Remember from Chapter 3 that there is a leaky gut connection that starts the whole autoimmune cascade? Gluten is one of the most common foods that contribute to leaky gut.

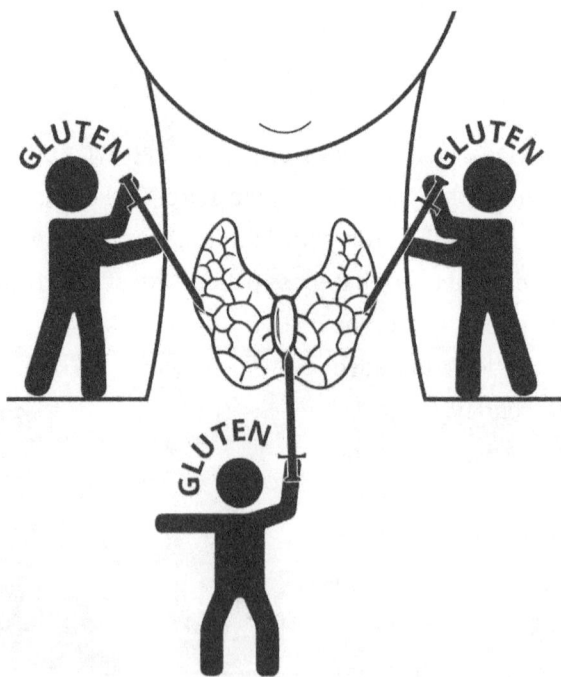

What Is Gluten?

Gluten is a protein found primarily in wheat, barley, and rye. When you go gluten free, you abstain from wheat, barley, and rye. Gliadin is the type of gluten found in wheat; hordein is found in barley; and secalin is found in rye.

Foods like rice, corn, amaranth, buckwheat, sorghum, oats, and other grains are technically considered gluten free, but these "pseudo-grains," just like gluten, can stress the immune system and cause inflammation and gut permeability.

They contain a high level of prolamin, which is a family of proteins within the grain family that gluten sits under. Prolamin proteins are high in the amino acid proline. Prolamin content can be high or low. Rice, for instance, has a 5 percent prolamin content, while corn has 60 percent.[2]

Antigenic load describes foreign substances or proteins that can elicit immune stress and inflammation in the body. It causes the gut to become even more leaky or permeable, which can increase the risk of an autoimmune condition. If you were truly going gluten free (recommended for those with a sensitive immune system or sensitive gut), you would cut out all grains and foods that contain cross-reactive proteins, like prolamin.

The Autoimmune Response to Gluten

The protein sequence in gluten looks very similar to that of the thyroid gland. If you're eating and consuming this inflammatory protein in grains and your body has a difficult time breaking it down, the gluten protein in the grain will eventually make its way into the bloodstream (gliadin and glutenin are the major protein components when describing gluten). When the protein gets into the bloodstream, the immune system sees that the protein can look similar to other tissues in the body (molecular mimicry), creating a case of mistaken identity (discussed in Chapter 3). In this case, the immune system starts sending out troops to attack that gluten protein.[3]

Since the gluten protein looks very similar to the thyroid tissue, the immune system mistakenly sees the thyroid as a suspect and also attacks it in the process, causing damage to the thyroid tissue. This is called an autoimmune response, when the body attacks itself. It was the gluten that kicked off the whole inflammatory reaction to begin with, but the thyroid is taking part of the punishment. It's like two children (gluten and the thyroid) getting in trouble for something only one child (gluten) did.

MOLECULAR MIMICRY

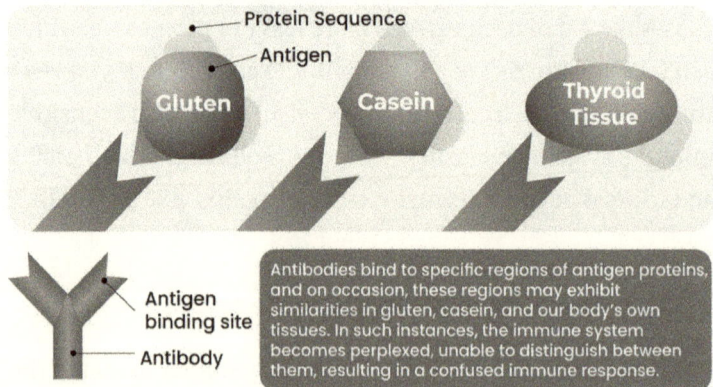

Protein Sequence
Antigen
Gluten
Casein
Thyroid Tissue

Antigen binding site
Antibody

Antibodies bind to specific regions of antigen proteins, and on occasion, these regions may exhibit similarities in gluten, casein, and our body's own tissues. In such instances, the immune system becomes perplexed, unable to distinguish between them, resulting in a confused immune response.

When these proteins have a similar shape to other proteins, cross-reactivity can occur. *Cross-reaction* is when the immune system starts responding to other proteins as if they were gluten. These proteins have the ability to bind other receptor sites, just like casein and gluten. As you can see in the following graphic, the shape of the antigen can be enough to confuse the immune system.

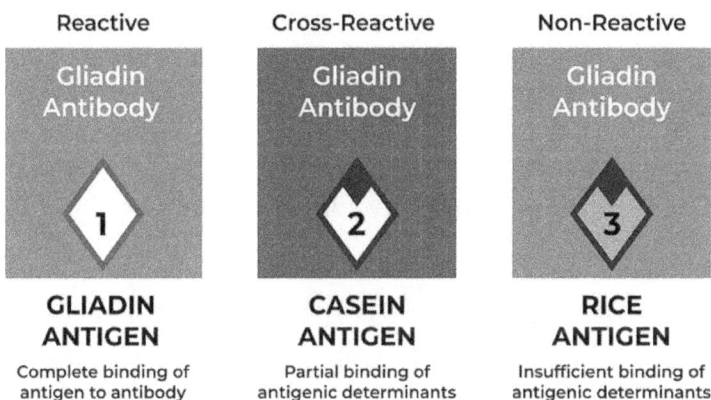

Reactive	Cross-Reactive	Non-Reactive
Gliadin Antibody	Gliadin Antibody	Gliadin Antibody
1	2	3
GLIADIN ANTIGEN	**CASEIN ANTIGEN**	**RICE ANTIGEN**
Complete binding of antigen to antibody	Partial binding of antigenic determinants	Insufficient binding of antigenic determinants

This is the reason why some people who remove only some grains from their diet but not all may not recover fully. The consumption of other cross-reactive foods outside of gluten can be enough to prevent your thyroid from healing.

We discussed earlier that up to 90 percent of Hashimoto's cases can be autoimmune in nature. According to Dr. Alessio Fasano, gluten is one of the top stimulators or triggers of leaky gut and, thus, autoimmune conditions.[4] According to Fasano's research, the Hashimoto–gluten connection shows that the antibodies and inflammation from consuming these grains can last up to six months in some cases. When you consume grains, the collateral damage can last for a short period of time for people who are less genetically susceptible. Think of it this way: every time you consume a little bit of gluten, imagine a piece of your thyroid burning up forever.

Only 1 percent of the population has celiac disease, yet this statistic is four to fifteen times higher when you have Hashimoto's.[5] I will say that again: up to 15 percent of all people who have celiac disease have a Hashimoto's autoimmune thyroid condition, not to mention up to 19 percent of all type 1 diabetics have Hashimoto's.[6]

Gluten Sensitivity and Celiac Disease

There is a small, specific sector of patients who have celiac disease, about 1 percent, while up to 99 percent of the population has a genotype that could make them susceptible to gluten sensitivity (HLA-DQ2 and HLA-DQ8 are celiac genes, while HLA-DQ1 and HLA-DQ3 subtypes are gluten-sensitive genes). In other words, most of us are sensitive to gluten. Only a small percentage of people with a genetic predisposition ever develop celiac disease though. This is partly because the disease diagnosis requires a significant amount of damage to be present intestinally for you to qualify. Also, epigenetic stressors, like poor diet and lifestyle, contribute to the genes expressing themselves in the first place.

I've observed that celiac patients who follow a gluten-free diet (eliminating wheat, barley, and rye) experience some health benefits. However, their condition significantly improves when they also avoid all grains and previously mentioned foods known to trigger autoimmune responses.

The issue with some gluten-free diets is that they often include alternative processed grains. These can still cause inflammation and lack essential nutrients that have anti-inflammatory properties.

When celiac patients went grain free, they healed significantly faster. This meant cutting out all grains (including those pseudo-grains discussed earlier), legumes, dairy, and even nuts, seeds, and nightshades in some patients. It took an autoimmune diet for them to really start healing.

There was a patient named Sally who came into my clinic years ago. Sally had all kinds of digestive symptoms (IBS), thyroid dysfunction (Hashimoto's), and eczema as well. She was really trying to get better as she was on a gluten-free diet, eating lots of oatmeal for breakfast, corn tortillas in the afternoon, and rice at night, and she was still having a difficult time healing. It was clear that she was still eating lots of grains. Once I got her on a grain-free, anti-inflammatory diet, her body started the process of healing. We had to address other hormonal imbalances and gut dysbiosis that were also present. We also needed to add in additional digestive support as she was chronically bloated and gassy after meals and was having a hard time digesting her food.

Celiac patients heal even faster when using the entire 6R strategy covered in Chapter 3:

1. **Remove** hyperallergenic foods
2. **Replace** enzymes, acids, and bile salts
3. **Repair** with healing nutrients, adrenal, and hormone support

4. **Remove** infections
5. **Reinoculate** with probiotics and prebiotics
6. **Retest** to make sure infection has cleared

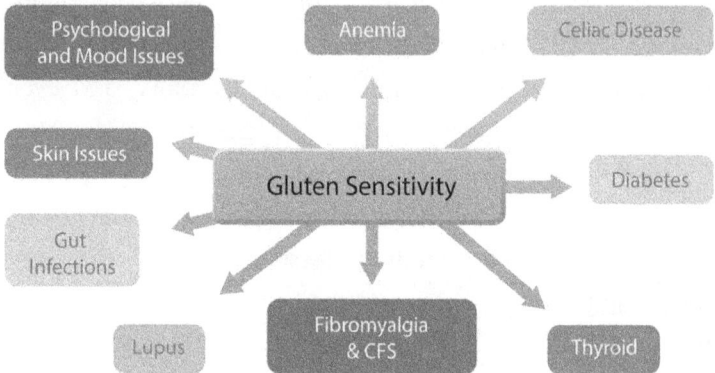

Symptoms of Gluten Sensitivity

The problem with gluten sensitivity is that the majority of symptoms that come from gluten are not necessarily correlated with digestive symptoms (gas, diarrhea, bloating, and constipation).

With gluten sensitivity, you are actually eight times more likely to have extra intestinal symptoms (symptoms not related to the gastrointestinal tract, like headaches, depression, brain fog, and fatigue). This is the main reason why gluten sensitivity is so easily glossed over today. Most patients with gluten sensitivity complain of two or more symptoms, such as those shown in the pie charts below.

There are many common manifestations of gluten sensitivity. I call this the *web of gluten sensitivity*. It includes various anemias, type 1 diabetes, Hashimoto's or other thyroid diseases, fibromyalgia, chronic fatigue syndrome, lupus, gut infections, skin issues (psoriasis, eczema, dermatitis herpetiformis), and psychological and mood disorders (schizophrenia, depression).

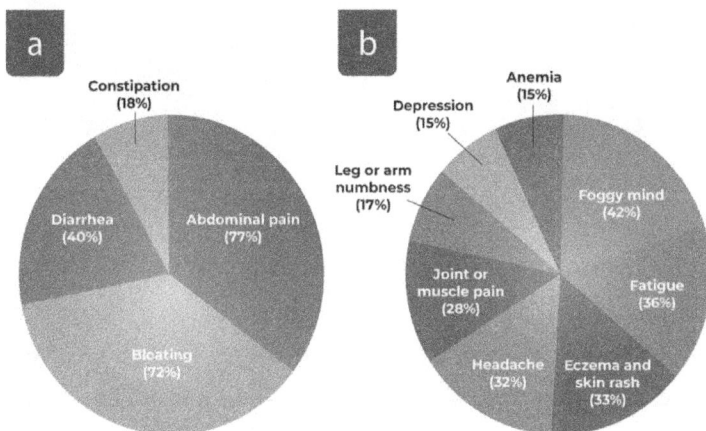

How Do We Know It's Celiac Disease?

Celiac disease is one of the most common autoimmune conditions and affects 1 percent of the population. One way we can tell if a patient has celiac disease is if they are making transglutaminase, endomysial antibodies, and deamidated gliadin peptide. These blood markers would be an indication of severe autoimmunity.

Another thing we look at is the *microvilli* in the small intestine. Microvilli are the vacuum cleaners of the small intestine. If they are clogged, they can't soak up all the minerals and nutrients you need to be healthy.

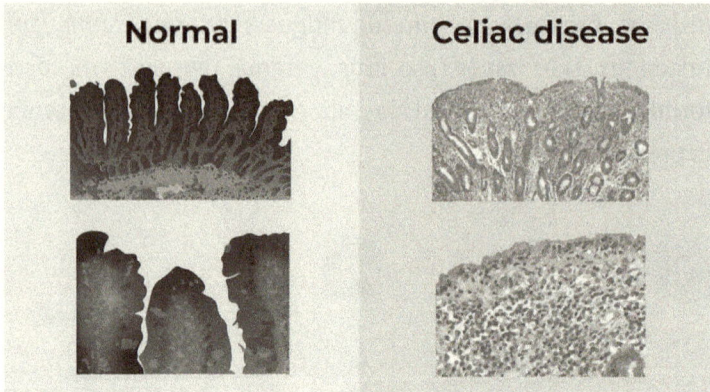

Normal   Celiac disease

Through an endoscopy, a doctor would go into the small intestine, take a sample of the microvilli, and look for *villous atrophy*, a wasting away of the microvilli. Many of these samples will show an increase in IEL (*intraepithelial lymphocytes*), which are essentially immune cells in your gut. When villous atrophy occurs at a level of 80 percent or higher, the diagnosis may be celiac disease rather than just a gluten sensitivity. Some may also use what's called a Marsh score, where typically a Marsh 2 would be indicative of celiac disease (Marsh 0 = long health villi, no celiac; Marsh 4 = flat, no villi, extreme celiac).

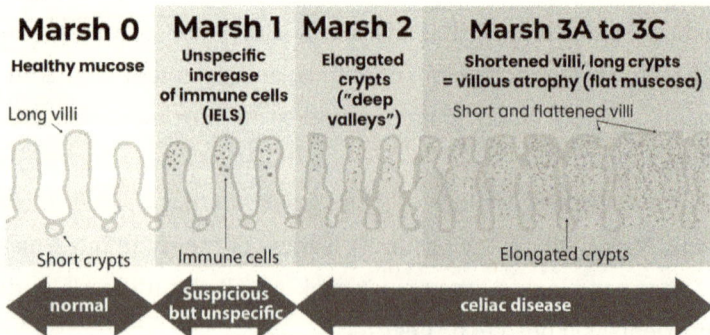

Marsh 0	Marsh 1	Marsh 2	Marsh 3A to 3C
Healthy mucose	Unspecific increase of immune cells (IELS)	Elongated crypts ("deep valleys")	Shortened villi, long crypts = villous atrophy (flat muscosa)
Long villi			Short and flattened villi
Short crypts	Immune cells		Elongated crypts
normal	Suspicious but unspecific	celiac disease	

There are hundreds of different autoimmune conditions. Celiac disease is just one manifestation of an autoimmune condition where the microvilli in the small intestine are affected. People who have celiac disease can have autoimmunity to other tissues in their body. Many of them suffer from *polyglandular autoimmune syndrome* (PGAS), where they have multiple autoimmune syndromes, and other glands become affected. For example, if they have celiac disease, they have a really good chance of having Hashimoto's, Lupus, Sjogren's, psoriasis, or rheumatoid arthritis, to name only a few. Where there's smoke, there's fire, and this is true for autoimmunity.[7]

Gluten Sensitivity, Celiac, and Genetic Testing

Gluten sensitivity and celiac disease have a genetic susceptibility associated with them, like most health ailments. The genes for gluten sensitivity or celiac disease, HLA-DQ2 and HLA-DQ8, increase your chance of having issues with gluten and grains exponentially. You get one gene from your mom and one from your dad; some people will have both genes, and some will have only one. Almost 95 percent of patients who have celiac disease have the HLA-DQ2 genotype, and the rest have the HLA-DQ8 genotype.[8]

HLA-DQ1 and HLA-DQ3 are the genes for gluten sensitivity. There are also subtypes, alpha 1 and beta 1, for gluten-sensitive individuals. This is important because if you are gluten sensitive, you still have a really good chance of reacting to gluten like a celiac, but you may never test positive for celiac.

Most people who have gluten or grain issues go to their conventional doctor, and the doctor runs the celiac tests mentioned earlier. He's looking for that villous atrophy and the endomysial and transglutaminase antibodies, but nothing comes up. Then he tells the patient, "You're just fine."

The reality is that the patient may be gluten sensitive, but these tests won't show that. Since we know gluten sensitivity is a matter of genetics, a genetic test tends to be the absolute best test to look for gluten sensitivity.

Genetic testing that looks at HLA-DQ2, 8, 1, and 3 subtypes to assess gluten sensitivity does not guarantee that you will have celiac disease, but if you want to evaluate your genetic risk, you can find the link in the resources section at the end of the book.

There are labs that will look at antibodies to gluten. Your immune system calls out certain soldiers to go in there and attack the gluten. The problem with this is that your immune system may not be able to call out those soldiers because it may be too fatigued, or your body may be creating inflammation that's more T cell based than antibody based. If your body is creating inflammation via T cells, the antibody test won't help. Looking at the genetic blueprint can be more reliable.

The Elimination-Provocation Diet

In my clinic, typically your first step is to do an elimination-provocation diet. Using a full autoimmune protocol, we cut out gluten and all grains for at least one month. We really want you to go not just gluten free, but grain free. When you are grain free, we typically see a significant improvement in symptoms, and most of the improvement tends to be extraintestinal. This means we see an improvement in symptoms other than digestive symptoms. The typical digestive symptoms that improve include diarrhea, bloating, gas, and reflux. Symptoms outside of the digestive system that improve include brain fog, achy joints, fatigue, low libido, dizziness, ataxia, hormonal issues, and PMS. Many people get better just by cutting out gluten. The reason why is because gluten is a strong inflammatory stressor on the body. The more inflammation and hidden stress there is in the body, the more the body has to deal with the inflammation via the adrenal glands, thyroid glands, liver, and detoxification system. The more stressed and taxed the body is, the more symptoms occur as a result.

By cutting out grains and doing a full autoimmune elimination diet for a month, most people notice a significant improvement. When they add the foods back in one at a time every two to three days, they may notice certain foods cause problems. Typically, doing an elimination-provocation diet tends to be the easiest and most cost-effective plan. Anyone who doubts it or is unsure may want to do a genetic test to rule out or confirm gluten sensitivity.

The Long-Term Effects of Gluten

If you have gluten sensitivity but continue to eat gluten, it's just a matter of time before other tissues become affected. You may have been able to handle gluten OK when you were younger, but as you got older and more things happened in your life that created stress and inflammation (sleep disruptions, infections, poor digestion, or emotional issues), your body may became more sensitive or reactive to it. Gluten may then break your body down faster and trigger autoimmune conditions because you're now susceptible to it.

Gluten Doesn't Bother Me,
So I Can Eat It, Right?

Let's say you can handle gluten. Let's even go a step further and say you're one of the rare few who doesn't carry a genotype for gluten sensitivity. It doesn't mean that gluten is doing no harm. Gluten can still cause inflammation and block mineral absorption.

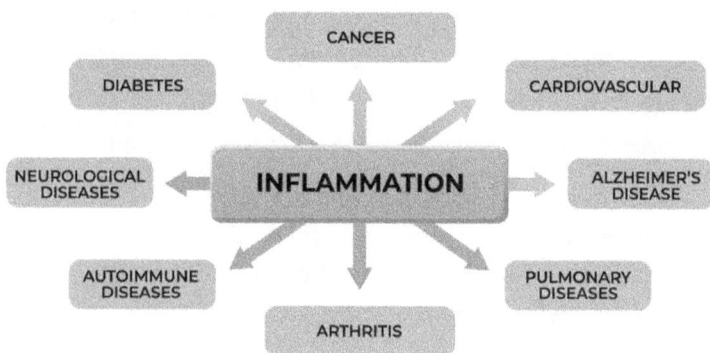

Why? First of all, gluten is inflammatory for one of many reasons because of a type of lectin (WGA) in it. WGA can make it harder to digest the gluten and create digestive intolerance symptoms like bloating and gas. It can also provoke the immune system to attack healthy cells.[9] It can cause inflammation in different people, and chronic inflammation can lead to a host of other diseases as you age.

Second, there are anti-nutrients like lectins, phytates, oxalates and trypsin inhibitors in grains which can impair protein, and nutrient absorption in grains, which are mineral blockers. This means the grains can also bind up minerals like zinc, calcium, and magnesium. Minerals are needed to manage stress and build strong bones, which is an excellent reason to avoid things that can potentially bind up minerals. This is why in many societies where only high amounts of grain are consumed, there's an increase in osteoporosis, bone weakening, and tooth decay. The more mineral absorption is impaired, the more nutritional deficiencies like magnesium are exacerbated, making it harder to grow and maintain healthy bones.[10]

The main genotype that isn't necessarily genetically sensitive to gluten is HLA-DQ4, but it is rare in America. Remember, the genes for celiac disease are HLA-DQ2 and HLA-DQ8, and the genes for gluten sensitivity are HLA-DQ1 and HLA-DQ3.

Of those with celiac disease, 90 to 95 percent have one copy of the DQ2 and DQ8 genes. According to Dr. Kenneth Fine, about 43 percent of the general population has either the DQ2 or DQ8 celiac genes, and another 38 percent has the DQ1 gene for gluten sensitivity.[11] Many of the remaining 19 percent have other gluten-sensitivity genes.

Genetic testing may show you are totally fine. Let's say you have the rare HLA-DQ4 gene. You still have the negative effects of mineral blocking and inflammation because gluten has wheat germ agglutinin in it. And grains typically don't have any special nutrients in them that you can't from other leafy green vegetables or safe starches.

Autoimmune Thyroid Disease and Gluten

If you have an autoimmune thyroid disease (AITD), you have to be very careful about gluten cross-reactivity, as discussed in "The Autoimmune Response to Gluten" section earlier in this chapter.

There is a link between Hashimoto's and gluten sensitivity. More clinicians are on top of testing AITD patients for celiac disease as of late. Also, the immune response to gluten can last up to six months from once you remove it from your diet.[12]

I have Hashimoto's, so I very rarely eat grains. If I have a serving of grain, maybe some steamed white rice that I'm confident is not cross-contaminated with gluten, it's a very small amount. Primarily, I'm 100 percent grain free with a small exception. When I typically cheat, I consume yucca- or cassava-based chips from the brand Siete. They taste really good and are 100 percent grain free; you just need to account for the extra carbs.

> Hashimoto's is a state of genetics; what we do have control over are the epigenetic triggers like diet, lifestyle, toxins, and gut function that allow the condition to express. Essentially, genetics puts bullets in the gun, and the environment pulls the trigger.

There's also a phenomenon known as *non-celiac gluten sensitivity*, which happens when people without celiac disease still have reactions, such as inflammation and gut permeability, driven by gluten exposure and the fermentable carbohydrates known as FODMAPs.[13]

Gluten and Stress

In Chapter 1, we discussed the Triangle of Health and the three stressors: physical, chemical, and emotional. With upward of 90 percent of the population having some degree of gluten sensitivity that they are overreacting to, it's just a matter of allostatic load (how full your stress bucket is). Your stressor could be blood sugar, sleep problems, nutrient deficiencies, poor diet, malabsorption, gut infection, poor stress management, or emotional stress at work, with friends, with family, or with your spouse, and then boom! Your stress bucket is overflowing.

Adding gluten on top of all the other stressors in your stress bucket may be more than your body can handle. Eliminating gluten is an important step in the right direction toward controlling stress.

The healthier you are, the better your chances of being able to tolerate some gluten here or there. I always tell patients that if you know you have an autoimmune condition, you always want to try to find a grain-free or at least a gluten-free alternative. It's just not worth the long-term inflammation if you are very sensitive.

Tests for Gluten

Outside of genetic testing, it's possible to look for antibodies in the blood and in the stool. Immunoglobulins G, A, M, and E (IgG,

IgA, IgM, and IgE) are antibodies that can show up elevated when testing for gluten, deamidated gliadin, or gliadin proteins.

Other more functional gluten tests will include different types of gliadins, wheat germ agglutinin, transglutaminase, glutenins, zonulin, and LPS (lipopolysaccharides) antibodies as well.

Unfortunately, there can be false negatives on these tests. Genetic testing can be a more reliable test to run to assess your risk of gluten sensitivity. This test is typically done via a cheek swab or blood test. However, antibody testing via the stool tends to be more accurate as the immune system is interacting with the gluten proteins more directly when they enter your gut.

Other inflammation markers that may be elevated from the collateral damage that gluten can cause are eosinophil protein X, lactoferrin, and c-reactive protein, and even liver enzymes like ALT or AST can be mildly elevated. Gluten isn't the only compound that causes these markers to elevate; that's why it is important to try an elimination diet as well.[14] When you feel better cutting food, that information is more valuable than any test. Especially if adding eliminated foods back in makes you feel worse, now you can be extra confident that the food is a problem.

The Conventional versus Functional Approach to Gluten

In individuals with celiac disease, gluten exposure can lead to severe harm. To be diagnosed with celiac disease, one must exhibit a high level of sensitivity to gluten, where even a small amount of grain can severely affect their health. It can take years for celiac disease to develop to a point where the damage is significant enough for a diagnosis. Traditional medicine often focuses on the late stages of diseases, prioritizing diagnosis and symptom management through medication and surgery. Consequently, many people suffer from symptoms for years before receiving a diagnosis of celiac disease. By this time, additional complications such as osteoporosis, digestive issues, nutrient deficiencies, and hormonal imbalances may also begin to emerge.

In individuals who are sensitive to gluten, gluten doesn't always act as a severe trigger. While it does cause a reaction and some inflammation, it doesn't lead to extreme illness. This is in contrast to those with celiac disease, who experience much more severe symptoms. People with gluten sensitivity might experience mild but persistent issues such as slight weight gain (around ten pounds), brain fog, premenstrual syndrome (PMS), fatigue, bloating, and gas. However, they often do not connect these symptoms directly to their gluten sensitivity.

Most conventional medical doctors will test their patient, get a negative result, and tell the patient that nothing's wrong; it's all in their head. These patients walk away under the false impression that gluten is OK to eat. In reality, the patient has just been ruled out of the conventional paradigm for a celiac disease diagnosis.

Gluten sensitivity is a functional diagnosis that is very real. But conventional medicine is so focused on pathology and disease states, which makes it very easy to miss. Gluten sensitivity predisposes many people to autoimmune disease, and given enough time and stress they may get there.

Conventional medicine is focused on the damage caused by the autoimmune condition. The problem is that the lag time can take years, if not decades. It's no fun to be one of those people sent home without an answer because there isn't enough damage to your body yet. The goal of this book is to let people know there are more sensitive markers and root cause solutions that can be used to help prevent years of damage and suffering.

Most people aren't aware, but 80 percent of your immune system is located in your gut. Following the 6R strategy mentioned below will give you the greatest chance to add more foods to your diet. Certain inflammatory foods like gluten and processed sugar are things you should keep to a minimum even if you can handle them every now and then.

Removing Hyperallergenic Foods in the 6R Strategy

Once the damage has been done in your body and you have a full-blown autoimmune condition, it takes a lot longer to heal. You can heal, but it takes a full dietary approach as well as getting the whole gut fixed. To go through this complete process of healing, you need to refer to the 6R strategy covered extensively in Chapter 3. Removing hyperallergenic foods includes gluten, and this needs to happen in step 1 of the 6R strategy. As a refresher, below are the 6 Rs:

1. **Remove** hyperallergenic foods (such as gluten)
2. **Replace** enzymes, acids, and bile salts
3. **Repair** with healing nutrients and adrenal support
4. **Remove** infections
5. **Reinoculate** with probiotics and prebiotics
6. **Retest** to ensure infection is cleared

Gluten-Free Backlash

Removing just gluten and grains may not be enough because you may suffer from "gluten-free backlash." I see many patients who will eat corn and rice—they may even be drinking sorghum beers—and they think they're doing themselves a big favor by going gluten free. But they don't get better because they aren't truly gluten free. They are still eating grains that keep them inflamed and impair mineral and nutrient absorption. They are suffering from a gluten-free backlash.

When I work with patients, I always feel the need to distinguish between gluten-free and grain-free anti-inflammatory diets. Technically, an apple is gluten free, but it is typically processed junk foods that get marketed as gluten free. Many people think they are doing themselves a favor by eating gluten free, but that also includes gluten-free processed foods, which can still cause inflammation. The grain-free, anti-inflammatory label is a much more accurate label and a higher bar to aim for. Also, eat most of your food from whole food sources, like vegetables, meat, and fruit; they don't come in packages.

You really want to abstain 100 percent from grains, legumes, and dairy; this is your typical paleo diet. I even go the full distance and eliminate other potential high-risk foods that can still be healthy for at least thirty days, including butter, nuts, seeds, eggs, and nightshades (tomatoes, potatoes, eggplants, and peppers). This is called the Autoimmune Paleo Diet (AIP). The goal of a diet like this is to eliminate all gluten and cross-reactive gluten foods, casein, the protein in dairy, and other foods that are high in anti-nutrients and lectins that can create inflammation in the body.

The autoimmune diet is not a forever diet for most people. We want to follow it for at least four weeks and wait until we see symptomatic improvements plateau for at least one week. Some patients see significant improvement even after thirty days, and I typically tell patients to continue on with the AIP diet until we see a plateauing of symptoms (no more improvements), then we follow my diet reintroduction handout when it's time to add foods back in. With some patients with known autoimmune conditions (RA, Lupus, etc.), we may maintain the diet for longer. You can access the diet reintroduction handout in the resources section.

Food Allergy Testing

Many conventional food allergy tests focus on measuring immunoglobulin E (IgE) levels. You might recall visiting an allergist and undergoing skin prick testing to determine if you're allergic to various pollens, dander, or grasses. You may also remember a classmate in elementary school who had a peanut allergy and needed to keep an EpiPen nearby. These are the immune reactions that conventional medicine typically examines.

However, we are more interested in food sensitivities, which involve immune reactions that are not as severe as full-blown anaphylactic reactions diagnosed by conventional medicine. There are other components of the immune system that can respond beyond the IgE response, including IgG responses and other T cell–mediated reactions.

The approach I find useful is the elimination-provocation diet, which involves removing potential allergens from your diet and then reintroducing them to observe any reactions that might indicate a food-related issue. It's important to note that these reactions can be extraintestinal, meaning they don't necessarily involve bloating or gas. Instead, they could manifest as fatigue, brain fog, or mood-related problems.

One reason I am not a fan of food allergy testing is that when someone has gut permeability issues, they are more likely to experience an immune reaction to any food they consume frequently. For instance, if you tested positive for a strawberry allergy and decided to replace strawberries with blueberries, it's highly probable that a retest in a month would show an allergy to blueberries as well. A useful principle to follow is "if you love it, rotate it." The more frequently you eat a particular food with a compromised gut, the greater the chance of developing an immune reaction to it.

That being said, there are high-quality food allergy tests available that examine more than just the typical IgG- and IgE-mediated reactions. At the end of this chapter, I will provide information on where you can find some of these specialized labs.

I have seen clinicians out there take the stance that these types of dietary changes are too restrictive for the patient and are setting the patient up for failure. My concern with this position is that you only have so much time to work with the patient, to gain their confidence, and to move their physiology in the right direction so healing can take place. If you don't make a drastic enough change, it won't push their body to heal fast enough, and confidence in the treatment plan drops, as does their compliance.

My position is that I always prefer to start the process with drastic changes that will produce rapid results that will then allow the patient to get more excited for the journey ahead. Based on my clinical experience, you don't have to celiac disease to benefit from removing gluten and grains. Also, the foods that we are adding in place of it are still far more nutrient dense, more anti-inflammatory, lower in toxins, and doesn't compromise gut permeability like grains can. There are not some magic nutrients in grains that we are missing out on, but we should choose other foods that have a better track record for promoting healing. I am always open to methodical reintroduction diet after a few months of stability. Expanding the patient's diet with other healthy foods is ideal.

KEY POINTS

1. Gluten is a strong agitator or stimulator for your immune system and can contribute to autoimmunity. It is one of the major foods that cause leaky gut.

2. Going gluten free is not the same as going grain free. Foods like rice, corn, amaranth, buckwheat, sorghum, oats, and other grains are technically considered gluten free, but these foods can cause genetically sensitive people a cross-reactive immune response.

3. Since the gluten protein looks very similar to the thyroid tissue, the immune system mistakenly sees the thyroid as a suspect and also attacks it in the process, causing damage to its tissue. This is known as molecular mimicry.

4. Everyone who has celiac disease is gluten sensitive, but not everyone who is gluten sensitive has celiac disease. Celiac disease requires more intestinal damage for it to be detected.

5. Gluten sensitivity and celiac disease are a matter of genetics. You either have the genes for gluten sensitivity or celiac or you don't. We have control of the triggers, exposure to gluten and grains.

Resources

Thyroid Reboot Foundations Bundle (www.justinhealth. com/foundations) Here are several recommended thyroid-supporting supplements mentioned in the book in easy-to-access bundles.

Diet Reintroduction Handout (www.justinhealth.com/diet-reintroduction) This handout will review the process by which I recommend adding new foods to my patients' diets.

Genetic Gluten Test (www.justinhealth.com/gluten-testing) This is a genetic gluten test that will test HLA for celiac disease and can be used to pick up gluten sensitivity. The markers include HLA-DQ2, HLA-DQ8, HLA-DQA1, and HLA-DQB1.

Celiac Disease Panel (www.justinhealth.com/celiac-disease-panel) This is a comprehensive blood test looking at immunoglobulin A, interpretation, and tissue transglutaminase. These markers are used to diagnose celiac disease.

Food Allergy Panel (www.justinhealth.com/food-allergy-panel) This is a more comprehensive food allergy test, looking at markers beyond your typical IgE or even IgG immune reactions. This will look at other immune reactions, including T cells.

Notes

1   David Yan and Peter. R. Holt, "Willem Dicke. Brilliant Clinical Observer and Translational Investigator. Discoverer of the Toxic Cause of Celiac Disease," *Clinical and Translational Science* 2, no. 6 (2009): 446–448, doi:10.1111/j.1752-8062.2009.00167.x.
2   Min Huang et al., "Quantifying Accumulation Characteristics of Glutelin and Prolamin in Rice Grains," *PLoS One* 14, no. 7 (July 18, 2019): 10220139, https://doi.org/10.1371/journal.pone.0220139; and P. C. Hoffman and R. D. Shaver, "A Guide to Understanding Vitreousness and Prolamins in Corn," University of Wisconsin–Madison, 2015, https://shaverlab.dysci.wisc.edu/wp-content/uploads/sites/204/2015/04/FGES-ProlaminGuidev2.0_000.pdf.
3   Aristo Vojdani, "Molecular Mimicry as a Mechanism for Food Immune Reactivities and Autoimmunity," *Alternative Therapies in Health and Medicine* 21, suppl. 1 (2015): 34–45, https://pubmed.ncbi.nlm.nih.gov/25599184.
4   Alessio Fasano, "All Disease Begins in the (Leaky) Gut: Role of Zonulin-Mediated Gut Permeability in the Pathogenesis of Some

Chronic Inflammatory Diseases," *F1000Research* 9 (January 31, 2020): 69, https://doi.org/10.12688/f1000research.20510.1.

5   Tejaswini Ashok et al., "Celiac Disease and Autoimmune Thyroid Disease: The Two Peas in a Pod," *Cureus* 14, no. 6 (June 23, 2022): e26243, https://doi.org/10.7759/cureus.26243.

6   Chin Lye Ch'ng, M. Keston Jones, and Jeremy G. C. Kingham, "Celiac Disease and Autoimmune Thyroid Disease," *Clinical Medicine & Research* 5, no. 3 (October 1, 2007): 184–92, https://doi.org/10.3121/cmr.2007.738.

7   George J. Kahaly, Lara Frommer, and Detlef Schuppan, "Celiac Disease and Glandular Autoimmunity," *Nutrients* 10, no. 7 (2018): 814, https://doi.org/10.3390/nu10070814.

8   Martina Sciurti, et al., "Genetic Susceptibility and Celiac Disease: What Role Do HLA Haplotypes Play?" *Acta Biomedica Atenei Parmensis*, 89 no. 9-S (December 17, 2018): 17–21, doi.org/10.23750/abm.v89i9-S.7953.

9   Karin De Punder and Leo Pruimboom, "The Dietary Intake of Wheat and Other Cereal Grains and Their Role in Inflammation," *Nutrients* 5, no. 3 (2013): 771–87, https://doi.org/10.3390/nu5030771.

10   Weston Petroski and Deanna M. Minich, "Is There Such a Thing as 'Anti-Nutrients'? A Narrative Review of Perceived Problematic Plant Compounds," *Nutrients* 12, no. 10 (2020): 2929, https://doi.org/10.3390/nu12102929; and Louise T. Humphrey et al., "Earliest Evidence for Caries and Exploitation of Starchy Plant Foods in Pleistocene Hunter-Gatherers from Morocco," *PNAS* 111, no. 3 (January 6, 2014): 954–59, https://doi.org/10.1073/pnas.1318176111.

11   Michele Sallese, et al., "Beyond the HLA Genes in Gluten-Related Disorders," *Frontiers in Nutrition*, 7 (November 12, 2020): 575844, doi.org/10.3389/fnut.2020.575844.

12   Elsa Mainardi et al., "Thyroid-Related Autoantibodies and Celiac Disease: A Role for a Gluten-Free Diet?," *Journal of Clinical Gastroenterology* 35, no. 3 (September 2002): 245–48, https://doi.org/10.1097/00004836-200209000-00009.

13   Giacomo Caio et al., "Effect of Gluten-Free Diet on Gut Microbiota Composition in Patients with Celiac Disease and Non-Celiac Gluten/Wheat Sensitivity," *Nutrients* 12, no. 6 (June 19, 2020): 1832, https://doi.org/10.3390/nu12061832; and Robert Krysiak, Witold Szkróbka, and Bogusław Okopień, "The Effect of Gluten-Free

Diet on Thyroid Autoimmunity in Drug-Naïve Women with Hashimoto's Thyroiditis: A Pilot Study," *Experimental and Clinical Endocrinology & Diabetes* 127, no. 7 (2019): 417–22, https://doi.org/10.1055/a-0653-7108.

14   Jaimy Villavicencio Kim and George Y. Wu, "Celiac Disease and Elevated Liver Enzymes: A Review," *Journal of Clinical and Translational Hepatology* 9, no. 1 (2021): 116–24, https://dx.doi.org/10.14218/JCTH.2020.00089.

6

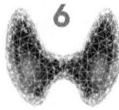

The Liver and Detoxification Connection

THE BODY IS ALWAYS DETOXIFYING. IT'S BUILT TO do this. The better question is whether or not detoxification is occurring at an optimal level? Are there additional toxins from your environment that are making it harder for your body systems to detoxify as well?

The liver's main responsibility isn't just detoxification. It also manages blood sugar and creates energy by converting the glucose or amino acids in the sugar via gluconeogenesis. The liver also makes important enzymes like the deiodinase enzymes, which are responsible for activating or converting T4 into active T3 thyroid hormone. This conversion process requires important nutrients like glutathione and selenium, which are also important for human health.[1]

The liver also filters out chemicals in foods during digestion that could cause stress. It is a major player in how the body functions. If the liver is not functioning properly, it will be impossible for the rest of the body to function optimally as well.

The Detoxification Process

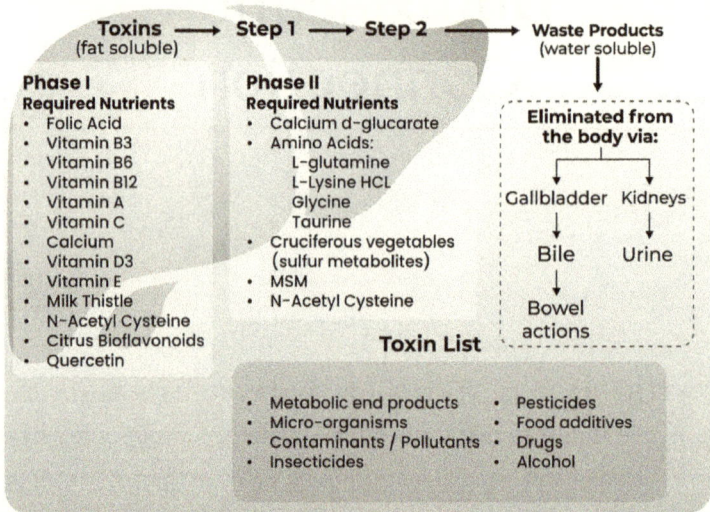

During detoxification, the liver interacts with the gut. A lot of the toxins that get pushed out of the liver travel from the liver into the gallbladder, and the bile that's concentrated in the gallbladder enters the digestive tract. Once in the digestive tract, the bile helps break down and emulsify fat-soluble nutrients like vitamins A, D, E, and K. We need fat to be optimally digested so we can absorb it. The bile is also bound up by the fiber from the food in your intestines, which is then eliminated via the stool.[2]

If you're interested in a blog post on detoxification to enhance this chapter, you can find the link in the resources section.

Detoxification Gone Wrong

If the digestive system is out of balance, constipation is a common symptom. Constipation is essentially slow bowel motility, and it shows up when you are unable to move stool through your digestive tract in a timely manner (typically twelve inches in a twenty-four-hour time frame). It can also manifest with difficult or incomplete bowel movement evacuation. It is usually caused by an unhealthy level of bad bacteria in the gut, infections, low stomach acid, biliary insufficiency, or low enzyme levels. Slow motility can also put additional stress on your liver.

If bad bacteria in your gut are elevated, enzymes like beta-glucuronidase can liberate toxins that were already bound up (conjugated). Another way to say this is that beta-glucuronidase can separate the toxins from the proteins that are there to escort the toxins out of the body. Instead of being eliminated, these toxins can now be reabsorbed into the bloodstream and wreak havoc on your body.[3]

This reabsorption through the gut causes major stress throughout the body, especially in the liver. The detoxification system primarily refers to the liver, but the liver interacts intimately with the gut. Without healthy gut function, the liver ends up having to deal with more stress because these toxins that had already made it through the gut now travel through the bloodstream and move right back up to the liver through the hepatic portal vein to go through the detoxification process all over again. It's as if the liver has to do twice the amount of work it usually does.

The Detoxification Pathways

When dealing with detoxification, the liver has three primary pathways.

1. **Phase I detoxification:** This is a nutrient-based pathway primarily involving B vitamins and antioxidants.

2. **Phase II detoxification:** This is an amino acid–based pathway and involves the transportation of the toxins out of the body. *Phase III detoxification* is sometimes used interchangeably with the elimination phase, Phase II.

Phase I Detoxification

Phase I detoxification is like putting food—some walnuts or almonds—down the garbage disposal. We're taking a fat-soluble toxin (in this case, nuts), and we're trying to make it water soluble by grinding it up really fine in the garbage disposal.

The goal of Phase I detoxification is to grind up these dense, fibrous compounds into something more liquid and water soluble in nature.

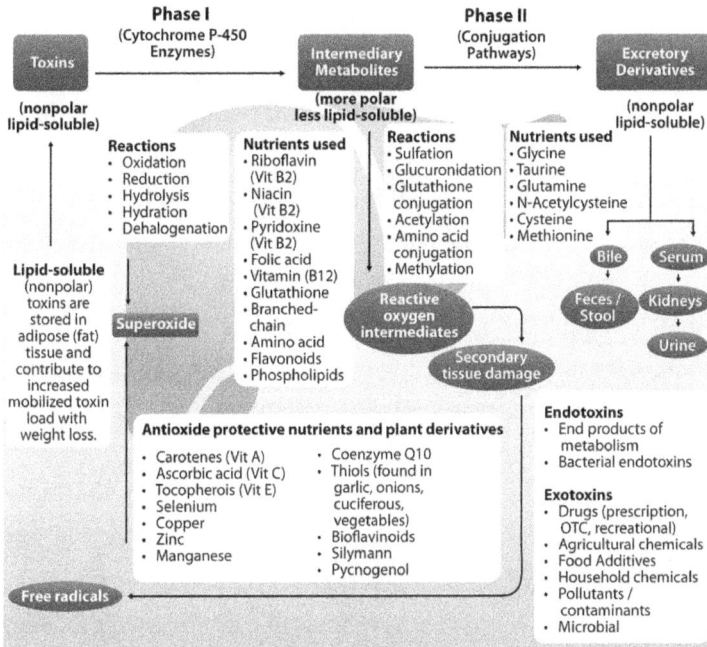

The chemistry of Phase I is called the *cytochrome P450 oxidase pathway*. Chemical reactions that happen in this oxidation phase include reduction, hydrolysis, hydration, and dehalogenation (the removal of chlorine, fluorine, and other halogens). Nutrients required to make these processes happen include vitamin B_2, vitamin B_3, vitamin B_5, folate, vitamin B_{12}, glutathione, branched-chain amino acids, flavonoids, and phospholipids.

Phase II Detoxification

Phase II of detoxification involves flushing out the compounds we ground up in Phase I. In Phase II, you are turning on the faucet and washing everything down the drain. You are taking these new water-soluble compounds and excreting them through the bile, into the feces, into the stool, and finally out of the body. Or they are being eliminated through the serum into the kidneys and out through the urine (also referred to as Phase III in some cases).

The chemistry of Phase II is called the *conjugation pathway*. Chemical reactions that happen in this phase include sulfation, glucuronidation, glutathione conjugation, acetylation, amino-acid conjugation, and methylation. The nutrients required to make these reactions happen include glycine, taurine, glutamine, N-acetylcysteine, cysteine, and methionine.

Problems in Phases I or II

If your body works through Phase I detoxification quite well but does not have an optimal Phase II, the pipes can still get clogged. After you grind up all those compounds, if they aren't flushed out, they'll solidify again and actually become more toxic. This gives us a clue to health: you really want to make sure you have all the nutrients in place for Phase II so you can flush out all the Phase I toxins. You don't want anything to stay behind.

It's really important that Phase II detoxification is working. A lot of people who are stressed or who have poor diets may not be getting enough of these sulfur amino acids to run Phase II. Or if you are vegan or vegetarian, you may not be getting enough complete, high-quality amino acids from your diet.

It's also possible that your body may be so toxic that it's using up all of these amino acids at faster rates, so they don't have enough amino acids left to run their detoxification systems optimally, and they may also have gut issues that are affecting their absorption.

If you are not breaking down protein optimally, it may be because of a gut issue, such as intestinal inflammation, infection, hydrochloric acid, or enzyme deficiency. If this happens, there's not enough protein absorption to run Phase II systems optimally.

The most important question about detox isn't whether you are detoxifying. To what degree are you detoxifying, and how toxic are you? If you're consuming a lot of toxins from your environment—from food, water, air, or hygiene products—then there will be more stress on your detoxification pathways.

Free Radicals and Detoxification

During detoxification, oxygen species known as free radicals can occur and cause cell and tissue damage. Because of this, it's imperative that antioxidants are present. The antioxidants keep free radical numbers under control. Antioxidants include vitamin A, vitamin C, vitamin E, selenium, copper, zinc, manganese, coenzyme Q10, various thiols, bioflavonoids, *Silybum marianum* (milk thistle), and pycnogenol oligomeric proanthocyanidins (OPCs) like grape seed extract and resveratrol.

Before and During a Detoxification Program

With Phases I and II of detoxification, it is important to also have healthy kidney function. This is why it's important to drink lots of clean water before, during, and after a detoxification program.

You also need healthy gut function, so before starting a detoxification program, make sure your gut is working appropriately and properly. This means infections have been knocked

204 · THE THYROID REBOOT

out. Go back to that 6R strategy in Chapter 3:

1. **Remove** hyperallergenic foods
2. **Replace** enzymes, acids, and bile salts
3. **Repair** with healing nutrients and adrenal support
4. **Remove** infections
5. **Reinoculate** with probiotics and prebiotics
6. **Retest** to make sure infection has cleared

The Toxins

Toxins can be anything from prescription drugs to pesticides, fungicides, molds and chemicals in your food supply. These toxins put stress on the liver and detoxification pathways. Toxins in pesticides found in food can also disrupt good gut bacteria and the gut lining. Toxins in metals can disrupt thyroid hormone production. Toxins commonly found in the environment that you may not be aware of include:[4]

- Phthalates, bisphenol A (BPA), BPA derivatives like BPS and BPF (which are similar) and other phenols mimic estrogen and conjugate thyroid hormones and eliminate them. They are found in plastics. This is why it's good to avoid plastics altogether.
- Polychlorinated biphenyl (PCB) is a pesticide found in various compounds, such as paints, coolants, and flame retardants.
- Glyphosate is the pesticide in Roundup that is sprayed on genetically modified (GMO) foods.

- Organochlorines—such as DDT, chlordane, or lindane— are found in insecticides.
- Metals—such as aluminum, arsenic, cadmium, lead, and mercury—can affect the thyroid.
- Mold is typically found in water-damaged homes or in homes with chronically elevated indoor humidity.

The Metals

Let's delve a bit deeper into the metals because they have such an impact on the thyroid. Every day, we are exposed to toxins like lead and mercury through coal, mercury fillings, certain fish, and industrial by-products. These metals have a known impact on increasing autoimmune attacks of the thyroid gland. Autoimmune thyroid conditions are the most common cause by which the thyroid gland becomes damaged and inflamed:

- Disrupt the production of thyroid hormones
- Inhibit T4-T3 conversion
- Provoke thyroid autoimmunity
- Disrupt the ability of the HPT (hypothalamus, pituitary, thyroid) axis or the ability of the brain to communicate with the thyroid gland

Metals are found in so many substances in our environment. Mercury, for example, is especially damaging to the thyroid because it can accumulate in thyroid tissue, provoking autoimmunity or making it worse.

Causes of Liver Stress

Inflammation can cause us to prematurely break down amino acids (such as methionine, lysine, or L-carnitine) that power the detoxification process, which can result in liver stress. This keeps our Phase II pathway from working properly.

Insulin resistance also causes liver stress by depositing sugar as fat in the form of palmitic acid in the liver, causing nonalcoholic steatohepatitis (NASH), or fatty liver disease. This can impede the liver's ability to regulate blood sugar. If the liver is under more stress, detoxification is going to be difficult.

Bad

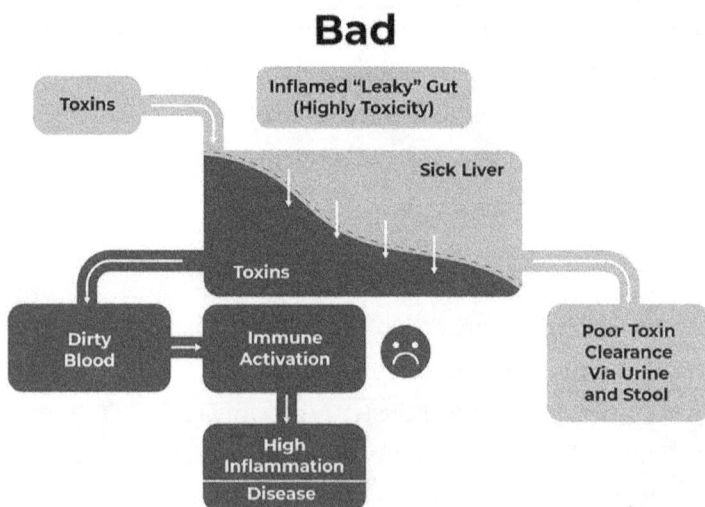

A leaky gut is also a big instigator of liver stress because it requires the liver to deal with additional reabsorbed toxins.

Imagine a dirty air filter in your house. The dirtier that air filter is, the more pressure and stress it puts on the air-conditioning unit. That's why you need to change your air filter every couple of months. A leaky gut is like an air filter that's dirty. And the liver is the stressed HVAC unit that has to handle the extra dust and debris and take on more of the burden.

How to Detoxify More Effectively

The best thing to do to more effectively detoxify is to stop exposure to toxins. This is the number one way. There are a number of ways to minimize and stop exposure, including eating organic food, avoiding plastics, drinking lots of clean water, and exercising.

Eat Organic Food

Eat food that doesn't have pesticides, fungicides, herbicides, or rodenticides and isn't genetically modified (GMO). GMOs contain glyphosate (the herbicide found in Roundup). Glyphosate is also a hormone and mineral disruptor. Disrupting minerals that are needed for detoxification minimize your body's detox efforts and prevent mineral absorption. It has also been shown to increase gut permeability (leaky gut). Minerals like selenium are very important for a healthy thyroid, optimal glutathione levels, and detoxification.

How do you know if your food is truly organic and non-GMO? At the grocery store, look for foods labeled with the "USDA Organic" green-and-white circle and the "Non-GMO Project Verified" tag.

You can learn more about the stringent standards that must be met to qualify for these labels on the following websites:

- USDA Organic: https://www.usda.gov/topics/organic
- Non-GMO Project Verified: https://www.nongmoproject.org

If you purchase from a local farm, ask the farmer if they use pesticides, rodenticides, or any other toxins on the crops. Farmers may not pay for the organic label, but they may still grow their foods based on organic practices. Having a conversation with your local farmer is a good way to find out what types of farming practices they adhere to.

There are other organic labels out there, but the standards to qualify for "organic" may not be strong. The USDA Organic label is a good certification. Some stores, like Whole Foods, will supply produce from local farmers, and they'll certify a food as 100 percent organic. Do your research and ask questions, though, because not all organic labels are created equal. Some farmers don't pay for the organic label certification but follow farming practices that are close to it, so it's always good to ask.

Eatwild, www.eatwild.com, is a good website for finding local farmers' markets near you to ensure that you get quality organic foods.

Avoids Plastics

Look for plastic products, especially those used in food preparation and storage, that are free from chemicals. Chemicals found in plastics include bisphenol A (BPA), phthalates, parabens, and other BPA xenoestrogen derivatives, such as bisphenol S and F (BPS and BPF).[5] Even if you purchase a bottle that is BPA-free, it will still have some of its estrogen-like derivatives that are not healthy for you. Drink from a glass bottle instead (my favorite brand is Lifefactory) or a stainless-steel canteen (my favorite brand is Klean Kanteen) instead of plastic bottles. If you typically buy bottled water in the store that comes in plastic, avoid stores that leave their plastic bottles on a loading dock, which exposes them to heat and UV sunlight, which increase the leaching of these plastic toxins into the water. If you need to buy bottled water in the store, shoot for a glass bottle brand like Topo Chico, Sanpellegrino, Gerolsteiner, or Mountain Valley. You can typically find these types of water brands at your local Whole Foods or natural health store.

Be careful of stores that don't have loading docks, like gas stations or convenience stores, as they more commonly leave their plastic water bottles out in the sun. If you drink out of plastic bottles, try to make sure it's less than 20 percent of your overall water consumption.

Drink Clean Water—Water Filtration

A whole-house water filter does a great job of filtering most toxins out of the water. This type of filter allows all water and showers to be usable with a significant reduction of impurities in the water. These types of filters consist of a pre- and post-filter as well as a large carbon filter, usually consisting of activated charcoal from charcoal or coconut shells. These filters can filter out residual chlorine, chloramines, parasites, bacteria, pharmaceutical medications, pesticide runoff, estrogenic compounds from plastics, and more.

A reverse osmosis under-the-counter filter is the best at filtering out all toxins. In a whole-house scenario, they are impractical due to the water waste they produce, but using them in your kitchen as a source of drinking water is a good move. Some will have a post-filter to add additional minerals back into the water. You can also use sea salt like Redmond Real Salt (just a pinch will do) or a high-quality trace mineral supplement to add some additional minerals back in. One of the many criticisms of an RO filter is that it can strip the water of all its minerals. My feeling is that it's best to have the cleanest water possible, as it's easier to add minerals back in than to pull toxins out.

Reverse osmosis filters typically consist of a number of semi-permeable membranes or stage filters (the more stages, the better) that the water is pushed through. As the water is pushed through these different membranes, all the minerals, including fluoride, and a higher level of all the contaminants mentioned above are filtered out as well. Typically, a whole house will filter out around 90 percent of most contaminants but will not touch most fluorides. An RO filter provides a great backstop as it will filter out everything else, including pharmaceutical drug residue that water treatment facilities do not filter out. In my house, I use both a whole-house filter and an RO filter system.

A countertop filter or water pitcher filter is an affordable option if you're not ready to make the above investment but still want to improve your water quality. Some of the filters above require changing your kitchen sink countertop or your water lines. If you don't own your own home, this may be an issue for you. A countertop system or water pitcher system is a great alternative as well. Some systems only make the water taste and smell better by removing chlorine; others will filter out more toxins. See the reference section in the back of the book for the specific products I use personally and recommend to patients.

Common Toxins Found in Water

Some of the toxins that can be found in water include fluoride, bromine, and chlorine. These are all included in the seventeenth group on the periodic table known as *halogens*. Halogens can disrupt healthy iodine metabolism, and you need healthy iodine metabolism to create thyroid hormone.

Fluoride is a major compound that can affect your thyroid hormone production. Fluoride is a halogen and fits into the same family as chlorine and bromine. There was a UK study in early 2015 that compared communities that fluoridated their water versus those that didn't. They found an increased incidence of hypothyroidism when the community fluoridated their water. The communities that had less fluoride in their water had less hypothyroidism.[6]

In the 1940s and 1950s, fluoride was used to treat hyperthyroidism. Doctors found that fluoride would slow thyroid function, easing the effects of an overactive thyroid. However, most of us do not have hyperthyroidism, so the overexposure we are getting to fluoride is damaging rather than benefiting your thyroid, potentially leading to hypothyroidism.[7]

16	17	18
		2 He Helium 4
8 16.0 O Oxygen	9 19.0 F Fluorine	10 20.1 Ne Neon
16 32.1 S Sulphur	17 35.5 Cl Chlorine	18 39.9 Ar Argon
34 79.0 Se Selenium	35 79.9 Br Bromine	36 83.8 Kr Krypton
52 126.9 Te Tellurium	53 126.9 I Iodine	54 131.3 Xe Xenon
84 209 Po Polonium	85 210 At Astatine	86 222 Rn Radon

Bromine is typically used in products like Mountain Dew and other sodas. It's also found in a lot of baked foods, grain products, and flame retardants. The flame-retardant *polybrominated diphenyl ethers* (PBDEs) are found in mattresses and other products, and a lot of kids' mattresses are mandated to have PBDEs in them. Young kids whose detoxification systems may still be developing and aren't working optimally are breathing in all these PBDEs, which can disrupt and interfere with thyroid production.

Chlorine is a compound that can be consumed and absorbed through the skin (e.g., while washing hands, swimming in a chlorinated pool, or taking a shower). It can become aerosolized, meaning you can breathe it in.

Chlorine is an antimicrobial that helps keep the water sanitized. I never understood why you would still want to consume even low levels of chlorine (1 ppm) based on its original purpose for being in the water in the first place. It makes sense to remove the contaminants when you are finally ready to use the water for bathing or hydration.

One area where a lot of bacteria live is your gut. Exposure to a lot of antibacterials, including chlorine, could potentially negatively impact your gut microbiome. Decreasing the amount of good bacteria in the gut can have a negative effect on the thyroid and the immune system.

Exercise

The skin can be used as a really good method of detoxification. Exercising and relaxing in a sauna, whether it's an infrared or near-infrared sauna, will help your body sweat out a lot of toxic compounds through the skin.

Liver and Detoxification Testing

Laboratory tests are helpful in finding acute toxin exposure. And typically, once you stop taking in a lot of toxic compounds, levels will start to drop on your tests. Liver and detoxification testing can be done via blood, urine, or even hair.

Organic Acid Testing

Organic acid testing can look at the metabolic function of your detoxification pathways. When we see imbalances in the organic acids that correspond with detoxification pathways, it's a sign that these pathways are either in high demand and are being burned up (like high RPMs on a car engine) or are being depleted due to increased metabolic stress (like low gas in the gas tank).

These acids tell us how Phase I and Phase II detoxification pathways are running and what nutrient imbalances may be present. Some of the organic acids included are:

- **2-methylhippurate**: Glycine or collagen peptides
- **Orotate**: Arginine, aspartate, magnesium, usually have a difficult time clearing your ammonia
- **Glucarate**: Glycine, glutathione, NAC
- **Alpha-hydroxybutyrate**: NAC, glutathione, taurine
- **Pyroglutamate**: NAC, glutathione, taurine
- **Sulfate**: NAC, glutathione, taurine

A test for pyroglutamate and 8-hydroxy-2'-deoxyguanosine can determine your antioxidant levels. The body needs not only

Phase I and Phase II nutrients but also antioxidants. Running the organic acid test can be very helpful to determine what is really happening in the body.

Proteins are needed to actually make organic acid in the body, so if you're having indigestion issues or digestive problems like low stomach acid, gut infections, and/or absorption issues, you may need to wait on running these tests until we can optimize amino acid levels and optimize digestion. Otherwise, we may get a false negative result on the test. These tests can give false negatives if you're not getting enough amino acids in your diet.

Urinary Challenge Test

Many people have a difficult time excreting the heavy metals that are in their bodies. This means that they will not necessarily show up in the test results. However, when a challenge test (also called a provocation test) is done, an accurate reading is obtained. In this type of test, a provocation agent is consumed. The test may be a simple urinary challenge test using a chelation compound. *Chelation compounds* remove heavy metals from the body. We use provocation agents such as DMPS, EDTA, or DMSA, and when we do this test, it's kind of like throwing a rock in a beehive.

Is the beehive empty, or is it full of bees? When the rock (our provocation agent) hits the beehive, the answer to this question will be evident within a second or so. If there are bees (heavy metals) flying out, there are a lot of heavy metals in the tissue that have been hiding in there. Giving a small dose of one of these chelation compounds gives us a window into what type of toxic metal load you may be dealing with. *Due to the risk of side effects, you do not want to use a chelation agent on your own. You should see a skilled practitioner for this.*

Many people can get into trouble by embarking on a full heavy-metal detoxification program without their hormonal, detoxification, and digestive systems working properly. When this happens, you can develop what's called a Herxheimer reaction, in which your body's detoxification, lymphatic, and immune systems are overwhelmed, thus making it harder to excrete these toxins. When you can't effectively remove toxins from your body, you end up reabsorbing them as they are now mobile in your body, creating inflammation and symptoms like extreme fatigue, achy joints, and flu-like symptoms.

If you have a healthy detox system, when your body provokes a release of heavy metals, you have the ability to run away and evade the bees and not get stung, as the analogy above depicts. It's not a big deal because you are healthy enough to deal with and adapt to the stress these toxins produce.

If you undergo a consistent heavy metal detoxification program without supporting an anti-inflammatory diet, hormone stability, good digestion, and motility, you have a great chance of feeling much worse. Detoxification of heavy metals is always one of the last things I focus on, as it requires a foundation of good health to engage in it successfully and not feel worse.

Hair Analysis Testing

Hair analysis testing can give false negative results with regard to heavy metal levels. You can use your hair as one of the many ways of detoxifying (including stool, urine, and even sweat). This means you can actually push metals out into the hair as a

216 · THE THYROID REBOOT

way for your body to reduce its levels of heavy metals. The idea for this test is that you may have a toxic level of heavy metals (mercury, lead, aluminum, arsenic, etc.) in your hair compared to what may typically be found in the average person. This gives us a window into your exposure level to heavy metals.

Where it falls short is that it doesn't give us a complete window into people who are having a difficult time detoxifying heavy metals. The fact that you can still push metals into your hair is a sign that you are still able to detoxify heavy metals at the cellular level. There are many people who are heavy metal toxic, with metals trapped in their tissues and organs that have reduced capacity for detoxification, allowing a false negative hair mineral test as their hair shows low or no heavy metal levels.

There have been studies looking at autistic children who were exposed to various levels of heavy metals, especially mercury.[8] They found autistic children had a difficult time detoxifying mercury through their hair when compared to children who were non-autistic, especially in the first few years of life. Hair mercury levels may be lower in a person when inefficient cellular mechanisms of elimination are present. Studies in monkeys show these heavy metals penetrate the blood-brain barrier and can stay in these organ tissues for months and even years.

Completing a urinary challenge test, both provoked (with chelation) and unprovoked (non-chelation), gives us a more complete picture of what someone's heavy metal tissue burden is.[9]

Blood Testing

Assessing heavy metals in the blood seems to be helpful only if the exposure to heavy metals is acute. If you ate some paint chips that contained lead in them in the last couple of days, you may see an elevation of lead in your blood. If you aren't getting exposed to a large dose of heavy metals on a day-in, day-out basis, this test will also give you a false negative. Most people's exposure to heavy metals tends to be at very low doses over a long period of time, where they bioaccumulate in the tissue.

Our bodies are very fastidious at keeping heavy metals out of the blood, where they can move around and damage tissues, create inflammation, and even damage neurons in the brain. The natural response is to move these heavy metals into surrounding tissues, especially fat tissue, where they are less mobile and less likely to cause damage and inflammation.

How to Start Detoxifying

Our body detoxifies better when the adrenals and thyroid have been supported (step 1, review Chapter 4), when the digestion is optimized (step 2, review Chapter 3), and when all the diet and lifestyle changes were made *before* undergoing a comprehensive detoxification program (step 3), whether it's a chemical detoxification or a heavy metal detoxification. It's also important to find a skilled functional medicine practitioner and get tested.

The Conventional versus
Functional Approach to Detoxification

Conventional medicine's approach to detoxification is to just abstain from the various toxins or drugs you may be addicted to. Or in cases of accidental poisoning like alcohol, for instance, charcoal binders may be used, and with overdoses of Tylenol, conventional medicine still recommends N-acetyl cysteine (NAC) to help detoxify the liver and bring up glutathione levels.

Conventional medicine's approach is more acute, meaning it's happening right now. In an alcohol or drug overdose situation, for example, they may pump your stomach or have you drink a cupful of charcoal water to immediately remove toxins from your system.

Conventional medicine typically uses three major blood tests to assess liver function:

- Alanine aminotransferase (ALT)
- Aspartate aminotransferase (AST)
- Gamma-glutamyl transferase (GGT)

When these enzymes are elevated, it can be a sign there is inflammation or damage to the muscle or organs. When there is an increase in ALT on a blood test, there is inflammation or damage to the liver occurring. When AST increases, there's a possibility of liver, heart, or muscle damage. And when there's an increase in GGT, there's gallbladder or bile duct inflammation or damage. These are the only tests that conventional medicine doctors typically use to assess liver damage or toxin exposure that affects liver function. There has to be quite a bit of inflammation and stress present for these markers to be elevated chronically, as in the example of an alcoholic with liver damage. It's possible to acutely increase these enzymes with a hard workout, as the breakdown of muscle tissue could give you a false negative as well.

For example, let's say a day or two before a blood test, you went on a bender and consumed a lot of alcohol. You may see a rise in ALT, AST, or GGT in your test results. I have also found that ALT rises due to increased sugar in the diet in those who have nonalcoholic steatohepatitis (NASH). Excessive fructose and high-fructose corn syrup intake can be a major stress on the liver. Exposure to the hepatitis virus could also cause an elevation in these liver enzymes, for example.

Avoiding toxins is the first step to lowering your toxic load, and that's why functional medicine practitioners emphasize the diet and lifestyle part first. Functional medicine goes above and beyond conventional medicine by emphasizing a higher-quality diet, one that's anti-inflammatory, nutrient dense, and lower in toxins. We also emphasize extra nutrient support to run your detoxification systems more efficiently and offer tests (covered under "Liver and Detoxification Testing" earlier in this chapter) that look at how your detox-ification systems are functioning. The functional medicine approach is ongoing—it's a lifestyle approach to ridding the body of toxins and minimizing intake so a major acute attack doesn't force you into acute symptom management with unnecessary drugs.

The Master Cleanse Trap

The master cleanse is typically a combination of a green tea, maple syrup, lime, and cayenne compound mixture. You sip on it throughout the day for a few days at a time. It is designed to help cleanse your body. The problem with this is that you're really not getting much nutrition from this cleanse. You need specific nutrients to run your Phase I and Phase II detoxification pathways.

In the master cleanse, you aren't getting the nutrients you need to run your detoxification pathways optimally. You're just getting a drink that provides glucose or sugar to stabilize your blood sugar levels, and it's also providing some hypoallergenic nutrients. Some people may report feeling pretty good while on it. The typical reason for this is that they are giving their digestive system a break because they are not taking in any solid food or any foods that have allergenic or inflammatory properties. While on a master cleanse, you are getting many of the benefits of fasting or intermittent fasting, which can help with recycling proteins (cellular autophagy), lengthening telomeres, helping with insulin resistance, and improving fat burning.

If you're used to consuming grains or foods that could increase inflammation, this can put stress on your gut and immune system and increase gut permeability. When you go on a master cleanse, you may feel better, but you're really not cleansing per se. You're not increasing your body's ability to detoxify—you're just lessening the inflammatory burden on your immune and detoxification systems.

The benefits of a master cleanse come from removing food allergens from your diet and giving your digestive and immune systems a break. People can get similar benefits sometimes by going on an autoimmune diet, and they won't lose the necessary nutrients to run their Phase I and Phase II detoxification pathways in the process. The people who do well on the master cleanse are those who have very tired digestive systems and a diet high in more inflammatory foods. The master cleanse could be a good transition on your way back to the healthier diet and lifestyle mentioned above.

While the master cleanse may be beneficial to some degree, don't get caught up in the master cleanse trap. Your body does need nutrients to efficiently detoxify toxins. Fasting, while it does have many health benefits, will not provide those nutrients.

Infrared Sauna Therapy

Sweating is a great way to push toxins from inside your body out toward your skin. The benefit of infrared sauna therapy is that it doesn't have to provide as much heat as a typical hot stone sauna. The infrared wavelengths penetrate deeper into the skin, raising the core body temperature and allowing a deeper level of detoxification from the body's fat layers beneath the skin.[10]

The key to an efficient sauna session is to come hydrated and even continue to hydrate with rich mineral water to prevent dehydration and low electrolytes during the session. You want to make sure you end your sauna session feeling just as good as when you started. A fifteen- to thirty-minute session can provide great benefits. Cut the length of your session down to an amount that allows you to feel equal to, if not better than, when you started the session.

You also want to make sure you don't forget to shower after the sauna session. Showering will help rinse all the fat-soluble toxins from your skin. Depending on the levels of toxins on your skin, I would use a 10 percent sulfur soap to ensure you are getting all of the toxins off your body. Regular soap is still good if that is all you have. The worst thing you can do after a sauna session is let your sweat dry on your skin and reabsorb all of those toxins again.

I find even my sensitive patients do well with infrared sauna therapy, and it's a modality that can be used early on even if your diet and digestion aren't fully dialed in. Just ensure good hydration, electrolytes, and a sauna session length that keeps you feeling good without any negative detox symptoms after. You can build up your sauna session length over time.

See the references in the back of the book and at the end of the chapter for my sauna recommendations.

KEY POINTS

1. The body is always detoxifying. But the more important question is this: Is your body detoxifying at an optimal level?

2. Mercury is especially damaging to the thyroid because it can accumulate in thyroid tissue, provoking autoimmunity and decreasing thyroid function.

3. Ways to minimize exposure to toxins include eating organic food and avoiding the use of plastics especially when heating foods.

4. The solution to pollution is dilution. Drink more water to help your body make toxins less toxic. Make

sure the water you are consuming is filtered, clean, and mineral rich. RO water filters will decrease fluoride in the water, which negatively impacts your thyroid gland.

5. Make sure you sweat! Adding infrared sauna sessions to your detox program can be helpful and is gentler for most sensitive people.

Resources

Thyroid Reboot Foundations Bundle (www.justinhealth. com/foundations) Here are several recommended thyroid-supporting supplements mentioned in the book in easy-to-access bundles.

Detoxification Support (www.justinhealth.com/detox) These are some of the detoxification-supporting supplements I recommend to my patients, ranging from sulfur amino acids and glutathione to liver-tonifying herbs.

Infrared Sauna (www.justinhealth.com/sauna) Here, you can find the specific sauna that I recommend to patients and that I personally use.

Organic Pasture-Fed Meats (www.justinhealth.com/meat) Here is a great site that sources grass-fed and organic food from Texas farms and can ship anywhere in the USA.

Organic Acid Test OAT (www.justinhealth.com/organic-acid-test) This test looks at organic acids, giving us a window into the function of metabolic processes in the body like detoxification, mitochondrial function, nutritional deficiencies, gut bacteria, and fungal overgrowth.

Urine Mold Testing (www.justinhealth.com/urine-mold-test) This test evaluates the mold toxins present in your urine. If your detox pathways are weak, using NAC or glutathione can help the body expel the mold toxins more effectively into the urine.

Environmental Mold Testing (www.justinhealth.com/environmental-mold-test) This is a mold plate test that can assess molds found in the environment, especially toxic molds that produce mycotoxins.

Environmental Mold Detox (www.justinhealth.com/environmental-mold-detox) This blend of botanicals can be used in a dry fogger as a safe way to help lower the mold in your environment.

Whole House Dehumidifier (www.justinhealth.com/dehumidifier) High humidity in your house can cause an elevation in mold. Decreasing your humidity with a dehumidifier can help decrease your mold levels.

Heavy Metal Testing Urine (www.justinhealth.com/heavy-metal-test) This test looks for heavy metals in the urine. It is typically used with a chelation agent to provoke a detoxification response.

Comprehensive Blood Test (www.justinhealth.com/comprehensive-blood-test) This is a comprehensive blood test that includes a CBC, metabolic panel, full thyroid panel, vitamin D, inflammation, and urinalysis. The metabolic panel includes liver enzymes as well.

Whole House Filtration (www.justinhealth.com/water-filters) This is a recommendation for the whole-house filter I use in my own home. This filter is carbon-based and has a pre- and post-filter for larger sediments as well.

Water Filtration Reverse Osmosis (www.justinhealth.com/reverse-osmosis) Here, you can find an under-the-counter reverse osmosis filter that I personally endorse. Reverse osmosis has the highest level of filtration.

Air Filtration (www.justinhealth.com/air-filters) Here is a high-quality air filter that I use with my family and recommend to my patients. This type of air filtration uses a HEPA air filter and an additional VOC filter that can filter other toxins typical air filters miss.

Sulfur Soap (www.justinhealth.com/soap) High quality 10 percent sulfur soap.

Notes

1   Antonio C. Bianco and Brian W. Kim, "Deiodinases: Implications of the Local Control of Thyroid Hormone Action," *Journal of Clinical Investigation* 116, no. 10 (October 2, 2006): 2571–79, https://doi.org/10.1172/JCI29812.

2   Daniel R. Schmidt et al., "Regulation of Bile Acid Synthesis by Fat-Soluble Vitamins A and D," *Journal of Biological Chemistry* 285, no. 19 (May 2010): 14486–94, https://doi.org/10.1074/jbc.M110.116004.

3   Yue Sui, Jianming Wu, and Jianping Chen, "The Role of Gut Microbial ß-Glucuronidase in Estrogen Reactivation and Breast Cancer," *Frontiers in Cell and Developmental Biology* 9 (2021): 631552, https://doi.org/10.3389/fcell.2021.631552.

4   Michelle Leemans et al., "Pesticides with Potential Thyroid Hormone-Disrupting Effects: A Review of Recent Data," *Frontiers in Endocrinology* 10 (2019): 743, https://doi.org/10.3389/fendo.2019.00743.

5   Syam S. Andra and Konstantinos C. Makris, "Thyroid Disrupting Chemicals in Plastic Additives and Thyroid Health," *Journal of Environmental Science and Health, Part C* 30, no. 2 (2010): 107–151, https://doi.org/10.1080/10590501.2012.681487.

6   S. Peckham, D. Lowery, and S. Spencer, "Are Fluoride Levels in Drinking Water Associated with Hypothyroidism Prevalence in England? A Large Observational Study of GP Practice Data and Fluoride Levels in Drinking Water," *Journal of Epidemiology and Community Health* 69, no. 7 (2015), https://doi.org/10.1136/jech-2014-204971.

7   Zohreh Kheradpisheh et al., "Impact of Drinking Water Fluoride on Human Thyroid Hormones: A Case-Control Study," *Scientific Reports* 8 (2018): 2674, https://doi.org/10.1038/s41598-018-20696-4.

8   Amy S. Holmes, Mark F. Blaxill, and Boyd E. Haley, "Reduced Levels of Mercury in First Baby Haircuts of Autistic Children," *International Journal of Toxicology* 22, no. 4 (July/August 2003): 277–85, https://doi.org/10.1080/10915810305120; Eleonor Blaurock-Busch et al., "Toxic Metals and Essential Elements in Hair and Severity of Symptoms among Children with Autism," *Maedica (Bucyr)* 7, no. 1 (January 2012): 38–48, https://www.ncbi.nlm.nih.gov/pmc/articles/PMC3484795/; David A. Geier et al., "Hair Toxic Metal Concentrations and Autism Spectrum Disorder Severity in Young Children," *International Journal of Environmental Research and Public Health* 9, no. 12 (December 2012): 4486–97, https://doi.org/10.3390/ijerph9124486; and M. D. Majewska et al., ""Age-Dependent Lower or Higher Levels of Hair Mercury in Autistic Children than in Healthy Controls,"" *Acta Neurobiologiæ Experimentalis* 70, no. 2 (2010): 196–208, https://doi.org/10.55782/ane-2010-1791.

9   Joseph Pizzorno, "Is Challenge Testing Valid for Assessing Body Metal Burden?," *Integrative Medicine* 14, no. 4 (August 2015): 8–14, https://www.ncbi.nlm.nih.gov/pmc/articles/PMC4712860.

10   Walter Crinnion, "Components of Practical Clinical Detox Programs—Sauna as a Therapeutic Tool," *Alternative Therapies in Health and Medicine* 13, no. 2 (March–April 2007): S154–56, https://pubmed.ncbi.nlm.nih.gov/17405694.

7

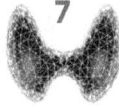

The Infection
Connection

NFECTIONS ARE NOT A PROBLEM FOR EVERYONE.
They tend to be more problematic for people who have weak-
ened or compromised immune systems. Simple diet and lifestyle stress can be enough to compromise your immune system
and make these infections a problem for you.

Autoimmune conditions like Hashimoto's or Graves' disease occur when specific antibodies are made by the immune
system to either attack or stimulate the thyroid gland. Certain
infections, when eradicated, may contribute to a significant
decrease in thyroid antibody levels (TPO ab, TG ab, and TRAb).
This means these infections can drive the immune system to
destroy the thyroid faster. If the infections are addressed—ideally naturally and safely—the killing and destruction the body

does to its own thyroid tissue can be reduced. This can then provide an opportunity for the thyroid to start healing.

If you have a compromised immune system and opportunistic bugs—parasites, bacteria, fungus, or viruses—come in and gain a foothold, that can create inflammation. That inflammation can create gut permeability, or leaky gut, discussed in Chapter 3, and impact your immune function. This can continue to perpetuate or exacerbate someone's dormant autoimmune condition. It can make it harder to digest, utilize, and assimilate nutrients from food. All of these bottlenecks in digestion can make it harder to deal with inflammation and detoxify the body. Each issue essentially compounds on itself, making it harder to heal and recover.

Typically, if someone is super healthy, that person can be more resistant to infections. The goal is to get people healthy by optimally managing their physical, chemical, and emotional stress (the Triangle of Health) so they have less risk of getting the infection in the first place. Lessening someone's infection load plays a major role in their journey back to optimal health.

TH1 versus TH2 Immune Balance

The TH1 and TH2 immune reactions represent two distinct methods that the body's immune system uses to combat infections and illnesses.

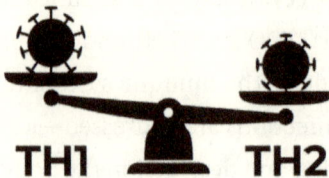

The TH1 reaction focuses on combating viruses and bacteria. It activates immune cells known as *helper T cells*

and *cytotoxic T cells* to eliminate infected cells and halt the infection's spread.

On the other hand, the TH2 reaction is responsible for fighting parasites and plays a role in allergic responses. It prompts the creation of antibodies and triggers other immune cells, such as B cells and eosinophils, to neutralize and remove parasites or allergens.

In a well-functioning immune system, TH1 and TH2 reactions collaborate and balance one another to provide effective protection against various threats.

When it comes to Hashimoto's, an autoimmune condition impacting the thyroid gland, this immune equilibrium is disturbed. From a functional medicine viewpoint, an unequal balance between TH1 and TH2 reactions can contribute to the onset and progression of Hashimoto's. If the immune system becomes imbalanced, favoring either TH1 or TH2 dominance, it may mistakenly target the thyroid gland, resulting in inflammation and compromised thyroid function.

Hashimoto's represents a TH1 dominant immune the majority of the time. The cytokines that represent TH1 are: IL (interleukin) 2, IL 12, TNFa (tumor necrosis factor alpha), and interferon.

TH2 dominance you would see includes: IL 4, IL 13, and IL 10. It's still possible for Hashimoto's patients to be TH2 dominant. You can run a cytokine panel to confirm.[1]

Hashimoto's could represent a TH1 or TH2 dominance, but there is research showing that it tends to favor the TH1 side.

The primary goal of the recommendations in this book is to identify and address the root causes of immune system imbalances. In this chapter, we discuss infections, which can significantly contribute to an unbalanced immune system from an infection standpoint. We have previously covered numerous essential nutrients that play crucial roles in maintaining immune balance, including vitamin A, vitamin D, curcumin, resveratrol, and glutathione. Other factors like gut inflammation, dysglycemia, cortisol dysregulation, and toxicity issues all play a role as well.

Compounds that stimulate the TH1 response:[2]

1. **Beta-glucans:** Found in the cell walls of fungi, yeast, and some bacteria, beta-glucans are known to boost TH1 immunity. These can be found in medicinal mushroom like reishi, cordyceps, maitake, and shiitake to name only a few.

2. **Echinacea:** A popular herb used in traditional medicine, echinacea has been shown to stimulate TH1 cytokine production.

3. **Astragalus:** A traditional Chinese herb known for its immune-boosting properties, astragalus may promote TH1 response.

4. **Medicinal mushrooms:** Various medicinal mushrooms—such as reishi, maitake, and shiitake—contain compounds that can support and stimulate the TH1 immune response. These also contain compounds known as *triterpenoids* that have antiviral and anti-inflammatory properties.[3]

Compounds that stimulate the TH2 response:[4]

1. **Vitamin C:** This essential vitamin is known to support the immune system and may stimulate TH2 cytokines.

2. **Quercetin:** A plant-derived flavonoid with antioxidant and anti-inflammatory properties, quercetin may promote TH2 immunity and also help break down histamine.[5]

3. **Licorice root:** Used in traditional medicine, licorice root has been shown to stimulate the production of TH2 cytokines.[6]

4. **Caffeine:** Found in coffee, tea, and other beverages, caffeine may have an effect on the immune system by promoting a TH2 response.[7]

Compounds with mixed or modulatory effects:[8]

1. **Vitamin A:** This essential vitamin plays a crucial role in immune system regulation and can have mixed or modulatory effects on TH1 and TH2 responses, depending on the context.[9]

2. **Vitamin D:** Similarly, vitamin D is essential for immune health and can modulate both TH1 and TH2 responses through the T regulatory cells, helping to maintain a balanced immune system.[10]

3. **Curcumin:** Found in the spice turmeric, curcumin has anti-inflammatory and antioxidant properties, and can modulate both TH1 and TH2 immune responses.[11]

4. **Resveratrol:** A natural compound found in red grapes, berries, and some other plants, resveratrol has antioxidant and anti-inflammatory effects, and can influence both TH1 and TH2 immune responses.[12]

5. **Glutathione:** As a powerful antioxidant, glutathione can help regulate the immune system and has modulatory effects on both TH1 and TH2 responses, contributing to a balanced immune response.[13]

Instead of attempting to manipulate the immune system in one specific direction using only these compounds, it is more beneficial to focus on uncovering the underlying factors causing immune stress and inflammation. By identifying the root cause of inflammation; supporting a healthy diet; addressing nutritional deficiencies, infections, and gut permeability; and ensuring the core nutrients mentioned above are adequately supplied, you help guide the body toward healing and finding its natural balance.

I Have a Bug, Now What?

You might be wondering to yourself, *Well, now that I have an infection, what's important to know and what do I need to do about it?* Infections tend to come from four major vectors:

people, pets, water, and food. Unless your symptoms come on strong right after an exposure (think drinking water from a stream while on a hike and getting diarrhea), it's difficult to connect the dots. In this section, I'll provide answers to these types of questions. First, the autoimmunity and infection connection.

The Autoimmunity and Infection Connection

The most common infections I see in my clinic are *Helicobacter pylori, Borrelia burgdorferi* (Lyme disease), *Epstein-Barr virus, Yersinia enterocolitica, blastocystis hominis,* and *Candida albicans.*

Helicobacter pylori (H. pylori)

As previously mentioned, H. pylori is a stubborn gram-negative bacteria that is common in over 50 percent of the population. Gram-negative bacteria contain a toxic compound known as *lipopolysaccharide* (LPS), and LPS is an *endotoxin*; it resides on the outer layer of the bacteria's cell wall. Getting exposed to H. pylori and other gram-negative bacteria can drive gut permeability because the endotoxin is a toxic stress on the liver and the enterocytes that make up the gut lining. H. pylori *can* also cause ammonia production, which has a very alkaline pH of 11. This shift in pH can negatively impact hydrochloric acid levels in the stomach, which are important for activating proteolytic enzymes like pepsin and digesting protein to name only a few.

Because gut permeability is an instigator of thyroid autoimmunity, it would seem logical that H. pylori's connection to leaky gut would also be connected to autoimmunity.

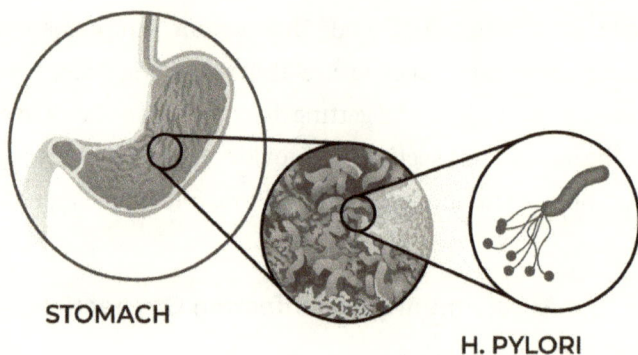

STOMACH

H. PYLORI

In one Italian study, two groups of patients, both with auto-immune thyroid conditions and H. pylori, were examined and some of them treated. One group was treated for the H. pylori infection, and the other group was not. They measured the antibodies in both groups from the start to the end of the treatment. There was a significant reduction in thyroid anti-bodies in the group that was treated for the H. pylori infec-tion compared to the one that wasn't. This was a profound finding because it showed that the infection had at some level impacted the immune system and exacerbated the body's immune response.[14]

So we know H. pylori is an infection that can potentially drive autoimmunity in the body, and when the infection is addressed, we see a reduction in those same thyroid antibodies. H. pylori is linked to other autoimmune conditions, too, such as multiple sclerosis.

Antimicrobials that could be used in treating H. pylori include berberine, oil of oregano, clove mastic gum, nanosilver, or other biofilm disruptors like ginger and N-acetylcysteine (NAC).

Borrelia burgdorferi (Lyme Disease)

Borrelia burgdorferi is a spirochete bacterium that is most commonly spread via a deer tick and can cause Lyme disease. The Borrelia amino acid sequence can look very similar to different parts of the thyroid tissue. There is research showing that Borrelia burgdorferi can exacerbate and drive an autoimmune attack of the thyroid tissue due to this similarity.[15] Other coinfections like *Babesia*, *Bartonella*, and *Ehrlichia* can also be found with Borrelia on deer ticks. This is why it is so important to test for other common coinfections if Lyme is ever suspected.

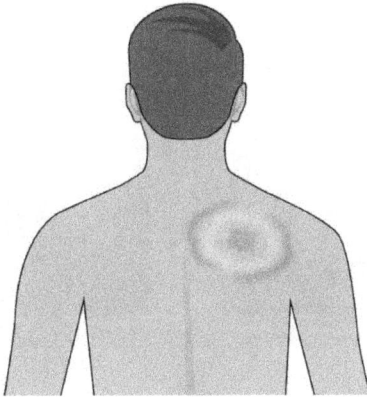

There are two types of Lyme disease situations: acute Lyme disease and chronic Lyme disease. Acute Lyme disease symptoms may include the classic bull's-eye rash on some occasions; a twenty-eight-day cycle of doxycycline is typically prescribed by your conventional MD to treat this infection, which may or may not address it. However, there are a lot of people with chronic Lyme disease whose disease has been festering for a long period of time. These chronic types tend to do better with certain long-term herbal treatments, as long-term antibiotic treatment protocols have a whole host of challenges that negatively impact beneficial bacterial levels in the gut. Natural compounds—such as silver, cat's claw, noni, berberine, goldenseal, neem, and medicinal mushrooms—are very helpful in supporting these types of infections.

Epstein-Barr Virus

Epstein-Barr virus (EBV) is the virus that causes mononucleosis. This infection is also known as the kissing disease. It is very common—80 to 90 percent of the population has had it. EBV can create an imbalance in the immune system where the *CD8-to-CD4 cell ratio* becomes skewed.

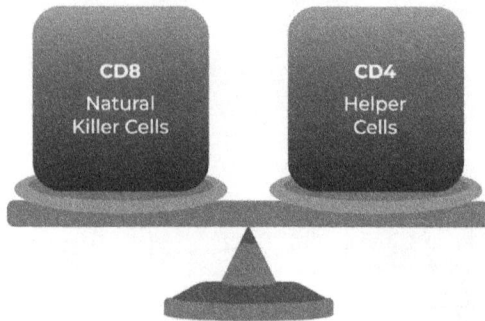

CD4 and CD8 cells are types of T cells that play essential roles in the immune system. CD4 cells, also known as helper T cells, primarily coordinate the immune response and activate other immune cells. CD8 cells, also known as cytotoxic T cells or killer T cells, directly target and kill infected cells or cancer cells.

The balance between CD4 and CD8 cells can influence the TH1 and TH2 immune balance. CD4 cells can differentiate into various subsets, including TH1 and TH2 cells, which have distinct roles in immune responses, as we mentioned above.

The natural killer cells—the CD8s—are like the Navy SEALs or special forces. They go in first and do all the reconnaissance and provide the intel, and they get things set up. They're the ones executing the attack right away. The helper cells, the CD4s, are the infantry—the marines, navy, or army. They're the ones waiting for the Navy SEALs to report back and let them know what's going on so they can come in and help out. If there's a CD8 deficiency, the first line of defense is much less than what it should be, while the CD4 (infantry) is much higher than what it should be normally.

Epstein-Barr is connected to many autoimmune conditions, such as myasthenia gravis, ulcerative colitis, rheumatoid arthritis, Hashimoto's thyroiditis, Sjogren's syndrome, multiple sclerosis, type I diabetes, and Guillain-Barré syndrome. Epstein-Barr also has a strong correlation to other immune diseases.

Women are four times more likely than men to have an autoimmune disease, and one primary reason they are more susceptible is because their estrogen levels can throw off the CD8-to-CD4 balance by causing a CD8 deficiency.[16]

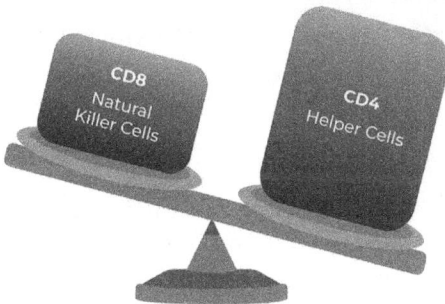

238 · THE THYROID REBOOT

Vitamin D, which is really a hormone, tends to be an important compound that can actually help with this CD8 T cell deficiency. Some of the nutrients we use to address EBV infections are vitamin D, selenium, medicinal mushrooms, chaparral, monolaurin, sulfur-based amino acids, and glutathione. Vitamin D is best received through the sun without burning, but for most people based on where they live, it would be nearly impossible to reach a therapeutic level. This is where supplementation would fill in the gap.

The Epstein-Barr virus can also be a trigger for chronic fatigue. Many people with thyroid problems report fatigue as one of their top three issues. It's important to rule out the Epstein-Barr virus if chronic fatigue symptoms aren't improving in the first three to six months of care. Other issues like poor diet, adrenal dysfunction, mitochondrial issues, low T3, gut inflammation, and poor nutrient absorption should always be ruled out first.

Yersinia enterocolitica

Yersinia enterocolitica is a bacterial infection commonly found in undercooked pork that can also trigger thyroid conditions and autoimmunity. It's found in food and contaminated water. As with the other infections, when this infection is eliminated, we tend to see a reduction in thyroid antibodies.[17]

Candida albicans

Candida albicans is a fungal infection that can cause many other issues as well. It can create malabsorption in the gut. The by-products of Candida are acetaldehyde and various mycotoxins that can put stress on the liver, disrupt digestion, create constipation, and cause motility issues. This can also throw off the gut flora, causing the dysbiosis discussed in prior chapters. There are other types of fungus similar to Candida that may also be present, including Geotrichum, microsporidium, and rhodotorula yeast. When testing for yeast, a stool sample can miss yeast or candida quite frequently. Using an organic acid test along with a stool test gives you a greater chance of catching it.[18]

Infections and Hormones

Gut infections can throw off hormones because the imbalance in the good-to-bad bacteria ratio (dysbiosis) up-regulates an enzyme called beta-glucuronidase. The body detoxifies hormones by conjugating them, meaning it binds them up so it can discard them out of the body via the kidneys, liver, or stool. The beta-glucuronidase enzyme prevents the protein from binding up the toxins. Imagine the toxic bacteria having a straitjacket around it. The straitjacket allows us to contain it so it can be escorted out of the body. When excess beta-glucuronidase enzyme is present, it comes in and unties that straitjacket, allowing the excess hormones to be reabsorbed. This results in more toxic stress being put on the body, creating a greater hormone imbalance.

Infection Tests

There are several tests that detect the different types of infections someone may have. These include blood tests, stool tests, urine tests, and breath tests.

Blood Tests

Lyme disease can be detected via a Western blot blood test, ELISA, or PCR (genetic-based testing). These tests can be run through various specialty labs.

Blood tests can also be used to detect Candida, Yersinia, Epstein-Barr virus, and H. pylori antibodies.

Stool Tests

Yersinia, H. pylori, and many other infections that can cause gut permeability (leaky gut) and exacerbate autoimmune conditions can be found on a comprehensive stool test by specialty labs. Most conventional hospitals or mainstream labs miss many of these infections.

The newer technology of stool tests involve using PCR DNA technology, which allows for testing a DNA fragment of a microbe and makes it thousands of times more sensitive.

I've had many patients come into my office who have already had conventional lab testing at Labcorp or their local hospital, and their test results have been negative. When the specialty labs are run, they are often positive for these various infections at a greater rate.

Breath Tests

A breath test can be very helpful in finding infections. A lactulose breath test can detect small intestinal bacterial overgrowth (SIBO). For H. pylori, a urea breath test measuring CO_2 is used.

A lactulose breath test is typically done over a two- to three-hour period. A baseline breath is taken first, and a lactulose solution is swallowed after. From that point, every twenty minutes, the patient will blow into a bag, where a QuinTron machine will measure the various methane and hydrogen gases that are present. This test can provide a good indirect assessment if bad bacteria are present by looking if excess methane or hydrogen gases are found. I personally prefer utilizing breath testing only if the stool and organic acid tests come up negative first.

The Conventional versus Functional Approach to Infection

Most people who see their conventional doctor do not get to the root cause of their thyroid autoimmunity. They're prescribed medications such as Synthroid, which may be necessary to bring down that elevated TSH. But one of the most common autoimmune drivers of elevated thyroid antibodies, H. pylori, can be frequently missed.

When conventional medicine does find H. pylori, they like to do a treatment called the triple therapy or quad that has a few different variations, including clarithromycin, amoxicillin, tetracycline, bismuth, and Prilosec (or other acid blocker) medication. This is typically a fourteen-day protocol, and many times it may not address the H. pylori infection due to antibiotic resistance. Also, there may be other infections present that the current medications have a difficult time eradicating, like other parasites, bacteria, and yeast.

In functional medicine, antimicrobial herbs or botanicals are used to help treat these issues. A number of these infections were addressed earlier in the chapter. As a refresher, a few of the antimicrobials used in functional medicine include the following:

- Berberine
- Oil of oregano
- Dill
- Grapefruit seed extract
- Mastic gum
- Matula Tea
- Silver
- Clove
- Barberry
- Goldenseal
- Slippery elm
- Wild indigo
- Wormwood
- Neem
- Ginger
- Thyme
- Samento or cat's claw
- Banderol

In functional medicine, the 6R approach is used to get to and treat the root cause of the infection. Removing the infection doesn't happen until step 4 of the process because addressing infections is stressful on the body. When people are stressed, there are usually multiple factors involved. Consider the following list of stressors and think about how easy it is to have additional stressors:

- Unhealthy gut bacteria or gut function
- Slow transit times
- Cortisol imbalances
- Hormone imbalances
- Low thyroid levels
- Poor lifestyle
- Poor diet containing a lot of inflammatory foods
- Difficult time staying asleep or going to sleep

When we knock out a bacterial or viral infection, the body has to deal with the dead debris. If someone is already dealing with the stressors mentioned above, killing and eliminating infections will potentially be enough to overflow their stress bucket, causing more symptoms to occur.

As the soldiers (the infectious organisms) start collapsing on the battlefield because of all the antibiotics, whether it's antibiotic medicines or antimicrobial herbals, the immune system, detoxification system, and lymphatic system have to send the medics out. These medics help pull soldiers off the battlefield. With so many soldiers on the battlefield, the medics get backed up. This backup is known as a die-off or Herxheimer reaction (discussed in Chapter 6), when all the biotoxins from the infectious debris accumulate and start creating immune stress, detoxification stress, and lymphatic stress. This is where it's common to feel tired, achy, foggy, and lethargic, to name a few symptoms.

The body has to be properly prepared to handle this stress and the infectious debris. Following the 6R approach in order will prepare the body's battlefield for victory.

Removing Infections Is Step 4 of the 6R Approach

When we are dealing with infections, the order of the 6R approach must be followed:

1. **Remove** hyperallergenic foods
2. **Replace** enzymes, acids, and bile salts
3. **Repair** with healing nutrients and adrenal support
4. **Remove** infections (good to check partner or spouse here as well)

244 · THE THYROID REBOOT

5. **Reinoculate** with probiotics and prebiotics
6. **Retest** to ensure the infection has cleared

This chapter has highlighted the fourth R: removing infections. Some of those natural antimicrobial medicines and herbs that help remove these infections can also kill beneficial bacteria, but they tend to be more selective for the dysbiotic bacteria than the good bacteria. The majority of the herbs we use are high in antioxidants, which can aid in reducing the oxidative damage from the killing process. Antibiotics, unlike clearing herbs, can increase oxidative stress in the body.

Have you ever thought about the comparison between your yard and your gut? Weeds grow automatically in your yard. No gardener will say they are going to Home Depot to pick up some weeds. Weeds just happen, similar to how infections occur in the gut. Once all the weeds are removed and cleaned out, there's a nice plot of land. It's all cleaned, tilled, aerated, fertilized, and ready to go. This is equal to removing the infection, and once that's done, we can throw down the seeds (step 5, reinoculating with probiotics and prebiotics) to crowd out any space for the weeds to grow and proliferate. The prebiotic fibers act like fertilizer to help the seeds that are being thrown take root more efficiently. More on this is coming up in Chapter 8.

Try Not to Self-Diagnose or Treat

You might be reading this book and saying to yourself, "Yes, I'm tired. So much of this sounds like me. I'm sure I have a thyroid issue. I probably also have a gut infection too."

It is very important to reach out to a skilled functional medicine practitioner who has experience dealing with thyroid issues and can look at all the other body systems and how they may interplay in your case. Try not to self-diagnose or use only the information provided here to self-treat. Many people get tunnel vision as they hone in on that one thing they think is wrong. It has to be mold, candida, SIBO, or Lyme. Many conditions have overlapping symptoms, and I always tell patients they have the right to have more than one thing going on at the same time. It's good to keep your mind open to all potential possibilities.

There are so many parameters and levels of health, and what seems like it can only be one thing may be something entirely different. Please seek the appropriate professionals who can handle your specific issues and set you up on an individual, customized plan. Sometimes very low cortisol may feel like low thyroid function, a B vitamin or iron-based anemia and sometimes the low cortisol may be driving the low thyroid function. It's important to find a practitioner who can gather information objectively and has a clinical framework that prioritizes all your

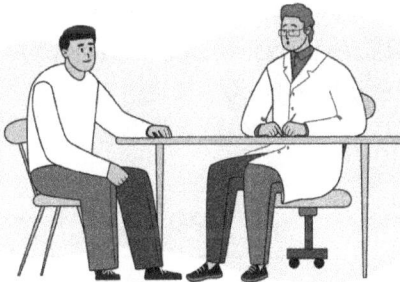

"I already diagnosed myself on the internet. I'm only here for a second opinion."

issues based on a best-practice order of priority. For example, we may start with diet, blood sugar stabilization, and foundational lifestyle issues first and then move up through the body systems. By the time you start going after bugs, you should have a solid health foundation underneath you. Yet time and time again, the opposite order, where bug and infection killing is addressed first, can cause a major setback.

Have you ever heard of people who choose to represent themselves in court? If they aren't a lawyer, their case very rarely ends well. There are many processes, motions, and terminology that if you aren't familiar with, you will get lost. The same thing happens in medicine and physiology. Not having the experience to assess what the root contributing causes are and develop a sequential plan to address them can create frustration and even make things worse. Seeking out an experienced functional medicine practitioner can help speed up your healing journey. If you were to climb Mount Everest, you would want an experienced Sherpa to help navigate you along the way. This helps give you the confidence that you are going to make it to the top and avoid getting lost or hurt. The goal of this book is to help you get as far in the healing process as you can on your own in a logical, sequential manner. Once you hit the wall, you know it's OK to ask for help.

KEY POINTS

1. When certain infections are eliminated, thyroid antibody levels can significantly decrease. This means

these infections could be driving the immune system to destroy the thyroid faster.

2. Leaky gut or gut permeability can be a primer for thyroid autoimmunity. Infections like H. pylori and other gut infections can increase gut permeability, thus increasing your chance for thyroid autoimmunity.

3. Borrelia burgdorferi causes Lyme disease and is most commonly spread via a deer tick; this infection looks very similar to the thyroid. Other Lyme coinfections should also be assessed.

4. Removing the infection should not be attempted until step 4 of the 6R approach because addressing infections can be stressful on the body (the only exception being acute food poisoning). Properly preparing the body (by doing the six steps in order) to handle the stress of the infectious debris is more likely to lead to victory on the body's battlefield.

5. It is very important that you reach out to a skilled functional medicine practitioner who has experience dealing with thyroid issues and supporting all body systems in a systematic way.

Resources

Thyroid Reboot Foundations Bundle (www.justinhealth. com/foundations) Here are several recommended thyroid-supporting supplements mentioned in the book in easy-to-access bundles.

GI Clearing Herbs (www.justinhealth.com/digestive) Here you can find some of the GI-clearing herbs that I use with my patients. These clearing herbs range from GI Clear 1 through 6, and they contain some of the herbs mentioned in this chapter.

Comprehensive Stool Test (www.justinhealth.com/stool-test) This is a genetic stool test that I recommend that uses sensitive PCR DNA technology that will detect bacteria including H. pylori, parasites, and fungal overgrowth. This test also assesses gut inflammation, immune function, enzymes, and fat malabsorption.

Lyme & Co-Infection Test (www.justinhealth.com/infection) This test looks at Lyme disease-causing bacteria and ten additional co-infectors. A positive result confirms DNA presence, while a negative result doesn't rule out infection. This test can offer clearer insights into Lyme disease and its related coinfections.

Matula Tea (www.justinhealth.com/h.pylori-tea) Matula Tea is an herbal blend originating from South Africa, traditionally used for its potential health benefits, particularly in promoting gastrointestinal health and as a natural remedy to help eradicate H. pylori infections.

Notes

1   Qiu Qin et al., "The Increased but Non-Predominant Expression of Th17- and Th1-Specific Cytokines in Hashimoto's Thyroiditis but Not in Graves' Disease," *Brazilian Journal of Medical and Biological Research* 45, no. 2 (December 2012): 1202–208, https://doi.org/10.1590/S0100-879X2012007500168.

2   Adrian F. Gombart, Adeline Pierre, and Silvia Maggini, ""A Review of Micronutrients and the Immune System—Working in Harmony to Reduce the Risk of Infection"," *Nutrients* 12, no. 1 (2020): 236, https://doi.org/10.3390/nu12010236.

3   Alena G. Guggenheim, Kristen M. Wright, and Heather L. Zwickey, "Immune Modulation from Five Major Mushrooms: Application to Integrative Oncology," *Integrative Medicine* 13, no. 1 (February 2014): 32–44, https://www.ncbi.nlm.nih.gov/pmc/articles/PMC4684115.

4   Gombart, Pierre, and Maggini, ""A Review of Micronutrients and the Immune System."

5   Yoshihito Tanaka et al., "Modulation of Th1/Th2 Cytokine Balance by Quercetin In Vitro," *Medicines* 7, no. 8 (2020): 46, https://doi.org/10.3390/medicines7080046.

6   Liiqiang Wang et al., "The Antiviral and Antimicrobial Activities of Licorice, a Widely-Used Chinese Herb," *Acta Pharmaceutica Sinica B* 5, no. 4 (July 2015): 310–15, https://doi.org/10.1016/j.apsb.2015.05.005.

7   Louise A. Horrigan, John P. Kelly, and Thomas J. Connor, "Immunomodulatory Effects of Caffeine: Friend or Foe?," *Pharmacology & Therapeutics* 111, no. 3 (September 2006): 877–92, https://doi.org/10.1016/j.pharmthera.2006.02.002.

8   Philip C. Calder et al., "Nutrition, Immunosenescence, and Infectious Disease: An Overview of the Scientific Evidence on Micronutrients and on Modulation of the Gut Microbiota," *Advances in Nutrition* 13, no. 5 (September 2022): S1–26, https://doi.org/10.1093/advances/nmac052; and Eva S. Wintergerst, Silvia Maggini, and Dietrich H. Hornig, "Contribution of Selected Vitamins and Trace Elements to Immune Function," *Annals of Nutrition and Metabolism* 51, no. 4 (September 2007): 301–323, https://doi.org/10.1159/000107673.

9   Mahdieh Abbasalizad Farhangi et al., "Vitamin A Supplementation
     and Serum Th1- and Th2-Associated Cytokine Response in Women,"
     Journal of the American College of Nutrition 32, no. 4 (2013): 280–85,
     https://doi.org/10.1080/07315724.2013.816616.

10   Maryam Soleimani et al., "Vitamin D3 Influence the Th1/Th2
     Ratio in C57BL/6 Induced Model of Experimental Autoimmune
     Encephalomyelitis," *Iranian Journal of Basic Medical Sciences* 17,
     no. 10 (October 2014): 785–92, https://www.ncbi.nlm.nih.gov/pmc/
     articles/PMC4340987.

11   Ming Zhang et al., "Curcumin Regulated Shift from Th1 to Th2
     in Trinitrobenzene Sulphonic Acid-Induced Chronic Colitis,"
     Acta Pharmacologica Sinica 27 (2006): 1071–77, https://doi.
     org/10.1111/j.1745-7254.2006.00322.x.

12   Lucia Malaguarnera, "Influence of Resveratrol on the Immune
     Response," Nutrients 11, no. 5 (2019): 946, https://doi.org/10.3390/
     nu11050946.

13   Serena Brundu et al., "Glutathione Depletion Is Linked with Th2
     Polarization in Mice with a Retrovirus-Induced Immunodeficiency
     Syndrome, Murine AIDS: Role of Proglutathione Molecules as
     Immunotherapeutics," *Journal of Virology* 90, no. 16 (2016): 7118–30,
     https://doi.org/10.1128/JVI.00603-16.

14   Giovanni Bertalot et al., "Decrease in Thyroid Autoantibodies
     after Eradication of *Helicobacter pylori* Infection," Clinical
     Endocrinology 61, no. 5 (November 2004): 650–52, https://doi.
     org/10.1111/j.1365-2265.2004.02137.x.

15   S. K. Singh and H. J. Girschick, "Lyme borreliosis: From
     Infection to Autoimmunity," *Clinical Microbiology and Infection*
     10, no. 7 (July 2004): 598–614, https://doi.org/10.1111/j.1469-
     0691.2004.00895.x; Devin D. Bolz and Janis J. Weis, "Molecular
     Mimicry to *Borrelia burgdorferi*: Pathway to Autoimmunity?,"
     Autoimmunity 37, no. 5 (2004): 387–92, https://doi.org/10.1080/0891
     6930410001713098; and Salvatore Bevenga et al., "Human Thyroid
     Autoantigens and Proteins of *Yersinia* and *Borrelia* Share Amino
     Acid Sequence Homology that Includes Binding Motifs to HLA-DR
     Molecules and T-Cell Receptor," *Thyroid* 16, no. 3 (March 2006):
     225–36, https://doi.org/10.1089/thy.2006.16.225.

16   Michael P. Pender, "CD8+ T-Cell Deficiency, Epstein-Barr Virus
     Infection, Vitamin D Deficiency, and Steps to Autoimmunity: A

Unifying Hypothesis," *Autoimmune Diseases* 2012 (January 24, 2012): 189096, https://doi.org/10.1155/2012/189096; and Vanessa L. Kronzer, Stanley Louis Bridges Jr, and John M. Davis III, "Why Women Have More Autoimmune Diseases than Men: An Evolutionary Perspective," *Evolutionary Perspectives* 14, no. 3 (March 2021): 629–33, https://doi.org/10.1111/eva.13167.

17 Zangiabadian et al., "Associations of Yersinia Enterocolitica Infection with Autoimmune Thyroid Diseases."

18 Iliyan D. Iliev and Irina Leonardi, "Fungal Dysbiosis: Immunity and Interactions at Mucosal Barriers," *Nature Reviews Immunology* 17 (2017): 635–46, https://doi.org/10.1038/nri.2017.55.

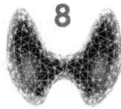

Nutritional Supplementation

NUTRIENTS ARE REQUIRED TO MAKE THYROID hormones. Back in Chapter 1, you learned about thyroid hormone conversion and iodination. Remember that *T4* is an inactive thyroid hormone made by your thyroid gland. *Iodination* is the process by which your body takes the amino acid tyrosine and binds it to iodine. When you see the number 4 next to T, the *T* stands for tyrosine, and the *4* stands for 4 molecules of iodine.

When we bind tyrosine to iodine, nutrients are needed to make it happen. Before we go over specific nutrients, feel free to access the nutrient counter app at the end of the chapter where you can log your foods for an average sample day. See the reference section at the end of each chapter. The app will give you a breakdown of the macro and micronutrients in your diet. This will give you a good starting point for determining what nutrients you should supplement or what dietary tweaks you can make to optimize your nutrient levels. Macronutrients (protein, fat, and carbs) can be addressed as well to optimize fat burning and insulin resistance. Most people with thyroid issues do well starting on the low-carb side, at least initially.

Nutrients Necessary for Thyroid Health

There are many nutrients necessary for thyroid health and thyroid hormone conversion. In this section, I'll share the most common.

Many of these baseline recommendations are based on the RDA (recommended daily allowance). Some people need higher levels than these, so it's important to get your nutrient levels tested to see if your nutrient demands are higher. It's always best to test, not guess!

It's best to review these recommendations with your functional medicine practitioner to see which you can optimize with food, and which may require supplementation.

Some people may find they still have nutritional issues even with a healthy diet. The next important step is to look at digestion and absorption and follow the 6Rs to address this issue.[1]

Iron

Heme based Iron, found in animal products like beef, liver, oysters, and salmon increase ferritin, the storage form of iron the

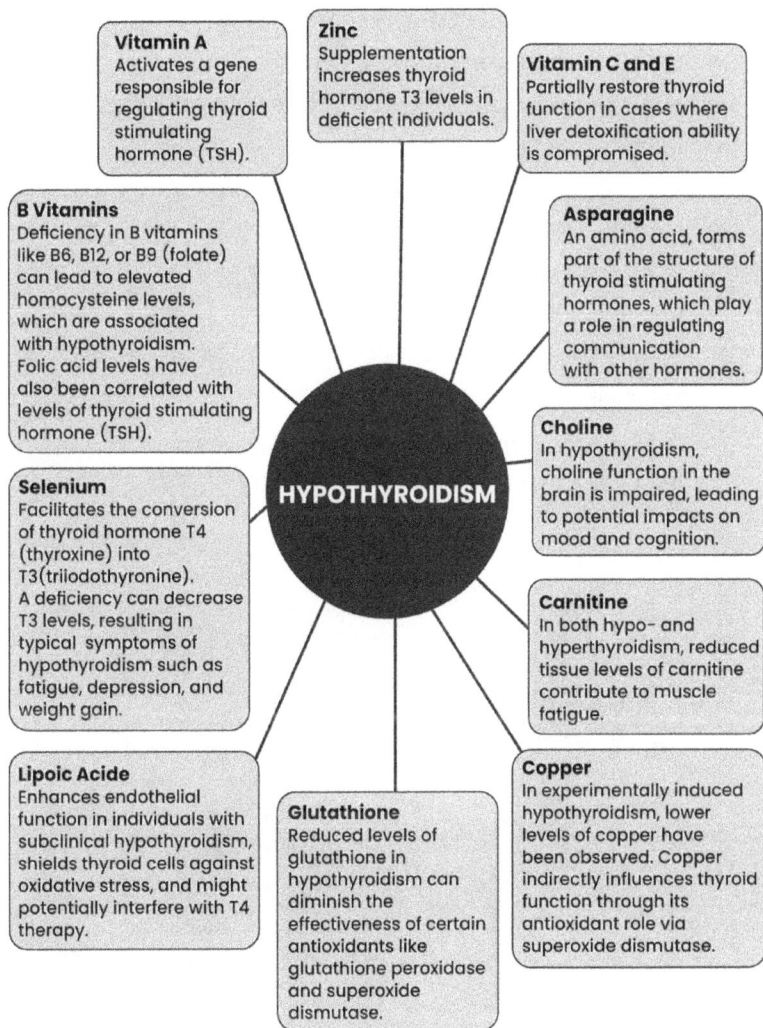

Vitamin A
Activates a gene responsible for regulating thyroid stimulating hormone (TSH).

Zinc
Supplementation increases thyroid hormone T3 levels in deficient individuals.

Vitamin C and E
Partially restore thyroid function in cases where liver detoxification ability is compromised.

B Vitamins
Deficiency in B vitamins like B6, B12, or B9 (folate) can lead to elevated homocysteine levels, which are associated with hypothyroidism. Folic acid levels have also been correlated with levels of thyroid stimulating hormone (TSH).

Asparagine
An amino acid, forms part of the structure of thyroid stimulating hormones, which play a role in regulating communication with other hormones.

Selenium
Facilitates the conversion of thyroid hormone T4 (thyroxine) into T3(triiodothyronine). A deficiency can decrease T3 levels, resulting in typical symptoms of hypothyroidism such as fatigue, depression, and weight gain.

HYPOTHYROIDISM

Choline
In hypothyroidism, choline function in the brain is impaired, leading to potential impacts on mood and cognition.

Carnitine
In both hypo- and hyperthyroidism, reduced tissue levels of carnitine contribute to muscle fatigue.

Lipoic Acide
Enhances endothelial function in individuals with subclinical hypothyroidism, shields thyroid cells against oxidative stress, and might potentially interfere with T4 therapy.

Glutathione
Reduced levels of glutathione in hypothyroidism can diminish the effectiveness of certain antioxidants like glutathione peroxidase and superoxide dismutase.

Copper
In experimentally induced hypothyroidism, lower levels of copper have been observed. Copper indirectly influences thyroid function through its antioxidant role via superoxide dismutase.

best. Iron is necessary for healthy red blood cells and oxygen transfer. The thyroid peroxidase enzymes that are involved in making thyroid hormone requires iron. Blood tests like ferritin, iron serum and iron saturation are good indicators of iron stores in the body. Symptoms of iron deficiency include the following:[2]

- Fatigue
- Shortness of breath with normal activities
- Pale skin
- Racing heartbeat
- Headaches
- Odd cravings: chalk, dirt, clay, and ice
- Weakness
- Brittle nails

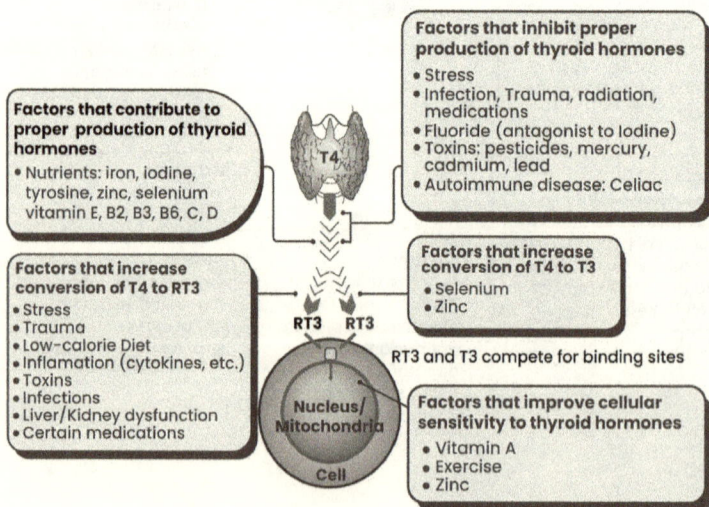

Factors that contribute to proper production of thyroid hormones
- Nutrients: iron, iodine, tyrosine, zinc, selenium vitamin E, B2, B3, B6, C, D

Factors that inhibit proper production of thyroid hormones
- Stress
- Infection, Trauma, radiation, medications
- Fluoride (antagonist to Iodine)
- Toxins: pesticides, mercury, cadmium, lead
- Autoimmune disease: Celiac

Factors that increase conversion of T4 to RT3
- Stress
- Trauma
- Low-calorie Diet
- Inflamation (cytokines, etc.)
- Toxins
- Infections
- Liver/Kidney dysfunction
- Certain medications

Factors that increase conversion of T4 to T3
- Selenium
- Zinc

RT3 and T3 compete for binding sites

Factors that improve cellular sensitivity to thyroid hormones
- Vitamin A
- Exercise
- Zinc

T4

RT3   RT3

Nucleus/Mitochondria

Cell

To boost your iron levels, try Iron Supreme, which is a highly absorbable iron chelate. Conventional iron supplements tend to cause constipation. A grass-fed beef liver supplement can also be helpful too.

Dopamine

Dopamine is a neurotransmitter. A neurotransmitter is a chemical messenger whose job it is to carry messages from one neuron to the next.

Dopamine is converted from its precursor chemical, L-dopa. The conversion can't happen without vitamin B6. Dopamine is essential not only to brain health but also to how the brain communicates with the thyroid (via the hypothalamus and pituitary) and to the production and conversion of thyroid hormone. Foods that stimulate dopamine production include eggs, fish, beets, and almonds.

- Below is a short list of dopamine deficiency symptoms:
- Feelings of hopelessness
- Self-destructive thoughts
- Inability to handle stress
- Anger and aggression under stress
- Desire to isolate oneself from others
- Unexplained lack of concern for family and friends
- Distracted easily
- Inability to finish tasks
- Need for caffeine to feel mentally alert
- Low libido
- Loss of temper for minor reasons

Recommended supplements

A high-quality multivitamin and tyrosine will help. Pure L-dopa from Mucuna pruriens can be more potent. With dopamine issues, important cofactors like B_6, folate, B_{12}, and a multivitamin are important to optimize neurotransmitter conversion. Healthy animal protein will provide the best food source of amino acids for dopamine.[3]

Iodine

Iodine is found in foods such as yogurt, seaweed, strawberries, tuna, eggs, potatoes, and shrimp. It's an essential building block for thyroid hormone. You may remember this from Chapter 1. Because a large percent of thyroid conditions occur due to an autoimmune issue, iodine can also trigger an autoimmune flare. It's important to have the right amount of iodine. A deficiency in iodine can lead to a goiter or thyroid nodules. Supplementing iodine when an autoimmune condition is present can increase inflammation and elevate thyroid antibodies. This risk increases particularly when selenium levels are low and other hormone and gut issues are present.

Too much iodine can cause a condition known as the Wolff-Chaikoff effect, causing short-term hypothyroidism. The thyroid gland responds to this extra iodine by shutting down thyroid hormone production for up to ten days as a protective mechanism.

On the other side of the fence, iodine can cause a condition known as the Jod-Basedow phenomenon, in which iodine causes the thyroid gland to go into a hyperthyroid state due to lack of feedback control from the pituitary. Iodine has also

been associated with many cases in the peer-reviewed litera-
ture of Hashimoto's thyroiditis.

TOP 10 IODINE FOODS

1.	Dried Seaweed		4500 mcg (100% DV) 1/4 oz	6.	Turkey Breast		34 mcg (23% DV) 3 oz
2.	Cod Fish		99 mcg (66% DV) 3 oz	7.	Navy Beans		32 mcg (21% DV) 1/2 cup
3.	Cranberries		90 mcg (60% DV) 1 oz	8.	Tuna		17 mcg (11% DV) 3 oz
4.	Yogurt		87 mcg (58% DV) 1 oz	9.	Strawberries		13 mcg (8.6% DV) 1 cup
5.	Baked Potato		60 mcg (48% DV) 1 MEDIUM	10.	Eggs		12 mcg (8% DV) 1 LARGE

Iodine can be a double-edged sword, and finding the right
balance can be tricky. This is why it is imperative that you work
with your functional medicine practitioner to determine the
proper iodine level for you.

If you have been diagnosed by a functional medicine doctor
and know you need to supplement iodine, Iodine Synergy is a
great option due to its addition of all the important cofactors
for thyroid conversion. Iodide doses between 150 mcg, which is
the RDA, and up to 1,000 mcg (1 mg) are a great starting point.
If iodine is added in, it's important to ensure thyroid antibodies are stable and other important mineral cofactors are present
like zinc, magnesium, selenium, etc.

Symptoms of iodine deficiency include the following:

- Goiter (enlargement of thyroid)
- Difficulty swallowing and breathing

- Choking sensation, especially when lying prone
- Hypothyroidism
- Depression
- Anxiety
- Fatigue
- Weight gain
- Trouble sleeping

Recommended supplements

Multi Support Pack, Thyro Replete, or Iodine Synergy in my supplement line are good options. If iodine is used, make sure antibodies and inflammation are stable. Start with the RDA of 150 mcg and gradually increase under your functional medicine doctor's supervision. Food options can also be used, but this can make dosing unreliable with seaweed food sources. Using kelp in supplement form may be the best option if using food sources.

Iodine testing

A twenty-four-hour urine test or an iodine loading test are the best to assess iodine levels. You can also complete an iodine serum blood test, which may provide less value, or an iodine patch test, which is the least accurate as most of the iodine is evaporated and not absorbed when painted on the skin.

Selenium

Selenium is found in meat, poultry, seafood, eggs, and Brazil nuts. It's an essential mineral that's necessary for thyroid hormone production. Selenium and cysteine are also responsible for the 5-deiodinase enzymes that are involved in pulling an iodine molecule off T4 and converting it to its active form, T3. Selenium and cysteine are also important cofactors for glutathione production, which helps with detoxification, immune function, and oxidative stress. In addition, selenium helps lower thyroid inflammation by converting hydrogen peroxide around the thyroid tissue into water, which can occur in the iodination process.[4]

TOP 10 SELENIUM FOODS

#	Food	Amount		#	Food	Amount
1	BRAZIL NUTS	544 mcg (100% DV) 1 OZ (6–8 nuts)		6	TURKEY (BONELESS)	31 mcg (44% DV) 3 OZ
2	YELLOWFIN TUNA	92 mcg (100% DV) 3 OZ		7	BEEF LIVER	28 mcg (40% DV) 3 OZ
3	HALIBUT	47 mcg (67% DV) 3 OZ		8	CHICKEN	22 mcg (31% DV) 3 OZ
4	SARDINES	47 mcg (64% DV) 3 OZ		9	EGG	15 mcg (21% DV) 1 LARGE
5	GRASS-FED BEEF	33 mcg (47% DV) 3 OZ		10	SPINACH	11 mcg (16% DV) 1 CUP

Symptoms of selenium deficiency include the following:

- Fatigue
- Hypothyroidism
- Irregular heartbeat
- Sensitivity to light
- Hair loss
- Low immunity defense
- Brain fog
- Reproductive issues

Recommended supplements

Multi Support Pack and Thyro Replete in my supplement line are good options. Aim for 200 to 400 mcg of selenium per day in a good, chelated selenium supplement like selenomethionine or glycinate blend.

Zinc

Zinc—found in foods such as meats, cashews, oysters, and lobster—is a required mineral for thyroid hormone production and conversion. Adding zinc as a supplement increases the T3 hormone in patients who have a deficiency. Symptoms of a zinc deficiency include the following:

- Fatigue
- Hair loss
- Low immunity defense
- Diarrhea
- Leaky gut
- Food and environmental allergies

Recommended supplements

Multi Support Pack or Multi Nutrient Supreme in my supplement line are good options. Aim for 15 to 30 mg per day in a good chelate, such as gluconate, citrate, picolinate, or glycinate.

Copper

Copper—found in foods such as oysters, liver, nuts, and seeds— assists iron in the production of red blood cells. Lower levels of copper are seen in hypothyroid patients. Copper indirectly affects thyroid status via an antioxidant called *superoxide dismutase*. Low levels of copper are associated with this antioxidant. Symptoms of a copper deficiency include the following:

- Fatigue
- Pale skin
- Hair loss
- Feeling cold
- Muscle and joint pain
- Weight loss

Recommended supplements

Thyro Replete in my supplement line is a good option. Aim for 500 to 1,000 mcg of copper per day in a good, chelated supplement like a glycinate blend, for example. Food sources are always best; filling in the gaps with supplements can help.

Glutathione

Glutathione is found in foods such as fresh and uncooked fruits and vegetables, grass-fed whey protein, eggs, and dairy. Glutathione is important, especially if you have low thyroid function, and is essential because it is a master antioxidant in the body. Glutathione is poorly absorbed, so it's best to use either a reduced, acetylated, or liposomal version for exogenous (outside source) supplementation. It's also smart to give your body the precursor amino acids so you can boost endogenous (inside source—your body makes them) production too. These amino acids include cysteine (NAC), glutamine, and glycine.

Glutathione cannot cross the blood-brain barrier, yet precursors like NAC can cross the blood-brain barrier. NAC can convert to glutathione while in the brain, aiding in neurological detoxification and inflammation reduction.[5]

Symptoms of a glutathione deficiency include the following:

- Weakness
- Headaches
- Dizziness
- Trouble sleeping
- Skin dryness
- Joint pain

Recommended supplements

Detox Aminos in my supplement line are a good option. Detox Aminos acids contain reduced glutathione as well as other precursor sulfur amino acids to help your body make glutathione as well. Aim for 100 to 500 mg of glutathione in either a reduced, acetyl, or liposomal version. NAC at 1 to 2 g per day can also help improve glutathione levels.

Lipoic Acid

Lipoic acid—found in foods such as organ meats, spinach, and broccoli—is an antioxidant and helps regenerate glutathione levels, and it helps stabilize blood sugar. Poor blood sugar levels—whether they are too high or too low—can affect thyroid conversion. Symptoms are similar to those of other antioxidant deficiencies and depend on the disease or disorder the person has. Lipoic acid can be used for heavy metal detox at higher levels as well.

Recommended supplements

I very rarely recommend lipoic acid by itself unless there are severe blood sugar issues or peripheral neuropathy.

Asparagine

Asparagine—found in foods such as plant proteins, meat, fish, and nuts—is an amino acid that is necessary not only for a healthy central nervous system but also for a healthy thyroid. Do you remember that TSH is really a pituitary brain hormone that talks to the thyroid, telling it to make thyroid hormone? Asparagine is essential because it helps with that communication from the TSH to the thyroid.

Symptoms of an asparagine deficiency include the following:

- Headaches
- Confusion
- Depression
- Irritability

Recommended supplements

I recommend food sources first. Individual amino acids can be taken if lab tests support low levels.

Carnitine

Carnitine—found in foods such as meat, poultry, fish, and milk—is made from amino acids, especially methionine and lysine. Its main job is to bring fat into the mitochondria and burn it for energy. Decreased carnitine levels can contribute to both hypothyroidism and hyperthyroidism. Imagine carnitine through a coal train analogy. To get the train to move, you would have to shovel coal into the train's furnace, where it would combust and create steam, which would then power the pistons, which would then cause the gears of the train to move. Carnitine is kind of like that, but instead of dumping coal into the engine and creating steam, fat is dumped into the mitochondria (the carnitine shuttle) where fatty acid oxidation occurs and adenosine triphosphate (ATP) is created, which can be used for energy in the body.

Symptoms of a carnitine deficiency include the following:

- Weakness
- Low blood sugar
- Cardiomyopathy
- Confusion
- Vomiting

Recommended supplements

Liquid Carnitine Supreme can be supplemented at higher levels to reach a therapeutic level between 1 to 5 g is good; too high can cause loose stools so be mindful and back off if you need to.

Choline

Choline—found in foods such as eggs, liver, cauliflower, and salmon—is an essential nutrient needed for proper mental function. Hypothyroidism negatively affects cholinergic function in the brain, which can affect mood and cognition.

Symptoms of a choline deficiency include the following:

- Memory loss
- Fatigue
- Muscle pain
- Mood changes

Recommended supplements
Aim for at least 500 mg per day. Individual nutrients can be taken if lab tests support low levels.

Other Nutrients Important for Thyroid Health

Vitamin A activates the genes that help support your thyroid-stimulating hormone (TSH), which helps prevent your brain from making too much TSH. Vitamin A also activates thyroid hormone receptors, so thyroid hormone can dock appropriately at the receptor sites. Vitamin A is a powerful antioxidant, has the ability to neutralize free radicals, and can also modulate T and B cells produced by the immune system. Vitamin A can also help lower autoimmune inflammation, which is the most common cause of thyroid issues.

B vitamin deficiency may elevate levels of homocysteine, an amino acid that can injure your cells and create inflammation. Low B vitamins are also linked to low thyroid levels.

B vitamins include the following:

- B_1 (thiamine)
- B_2 (riboflavin)
- B_3 (niacin)
- B_5 (pantothenic acid)

- B_6 (pyridoxal 5'-phosphate)
- B_7 (biotin)
- B_9 (folate, calcium folinate, or L-5-MTHF)
- B_{12} (as methyl, adenosyl, or hydroxocobalamin)
- PABA (para-aminobenzoic acid)

Vitamins C and E are actually antioxidants that help support the liver. A lot of thyroid activation and conversion happens in the liver, which requires good levels of vitamins C and E.

Vitamin D is actually not a vitamin but a hormone. The body produces it when sunlight touches your skin. Vitamin D helps balance the immune system and reduces inflammation. If you live in geographical areas where there's little sun or it's a season when sunlight is low, the body cannot make proper amounts of vitamin D. If you don't get enough sunlight, then supplementation is necessary. Supplement vitamin D around 5,000 to 10,000 IU per day, depending on size. As a good starting point, shoot for a vitamin D level at or greater than 50 ng/ml. With autoimmune disease, shoot for 60 to 90 ng/ml. You can retest your 25-hydroxy vitamin D via a blood test every two to three months to ensure you aren't taking too much. Vitamin D can be taken with K2 if you aren't getting enough in your diet via egg yolks, grass-fed butter, liver, and leafy-green vegetables.

Deficiencies in any of these nutrients can lead to hypothyroidism or other thyroid disorders. (Try the supplement called Multi Nutrient Supreme in my line for a daily boost of vitamin A, vitamins B_6 and B_{12}, vitamin C, vitamin D, and vitamin E plus zinc, iodine, selenium, and more!)

Nutrient-Deficiency Tests

There are a number of ways to assess nutrient levels, including the zinc tally test and assessing physical symptoms like fingernail ridging. There are different functional nutrient tests that can be used to detect nutrient deficiencies more specifically. Links to access these will be at the end of the chapter.

Zinc Tally Test

To determine zinc levels, a zinc tally test can be run. This is a taste test. You consume a tablespoon of zinc sulfate and closely observe the taste. The more neutral or even better the zinc sulfate tastes to you, the more deficient in zinc you are. The worse it tastes, or the more bitter or metallic it tastes, the less deficient you are. Your body indirectly tells you through your taste sensations what your zinc levels are. This is a cost-effective option to gauge whether you need additional zinc supplementation or if you should just focus on getting extra through your diet. Foods like seafood tend to be excellent, nutrient-dense options for zinc. One oyster contains 10 mg of zinc.

Fingernail Ridging

Your fingernails hold the key to many diseases and disorders. Ridging on the fingernails can mean a protein deficiency; you're just not getting enough protein. It could also mean you're not digesting proteins well. For any nutrient deficiencies, we always want to look at the gut

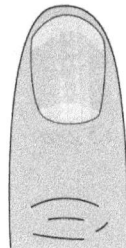

first. You could have a great diet and be taking great nutrients, but if there's a gut issue—malabsorption, leaky gut, infections, and so on—all the best supplements may not be enough.

Micronutrient Deficiency Testing

There are micronutrient deficiency tests that look at isolating the lymphocyte—part of the white blood cells in the blood—and essentially are able to detect various nutrient deficiencies by allowing these lymphocytes to grow in a controlled environment while isolating out thirty-one different nutrients. If the white blood cells have a slower growth rate in the culture while isolating selenium, then a functional deficiency with selenium exists. If the white blood cells grow well where vitamin A is isolated, that's a sign that vitamin A levels are sufficient. The rate at which the white blood cells grow indicates how sufficient or deficient one is in that nutrient.

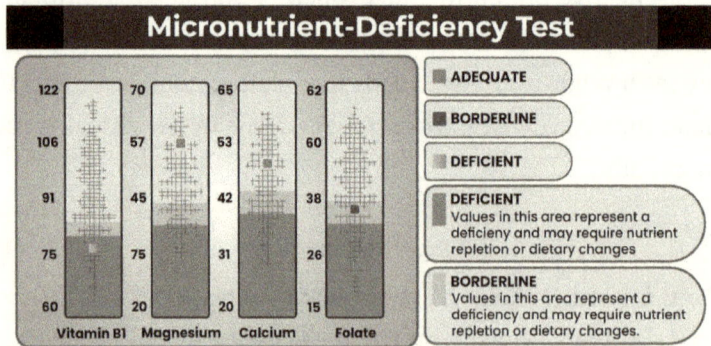

Organic Acid Testing

Organic acid tests basically look at the organic acids in the urine. Organic acids are the metabolites from the body that utilize amino acids or proteins for different body processes like energy production, detoxification, neurotransmitters, methylation, etc. Organic acids become metabolized when adequate levels of certain nutrients are present, specific to each metabolic pathway. If certain organic acids go high, the nutrients needed to metabolize the organic acids are low.

Imagine you have organic acid A. Organic acid A (methylmalonic acid) gets metabolized to organic acid B (succinic acid)—let's say in this example, by the nutrient B_{12}. If organic acid A stays high and B stays really low, that means A is not being metabolized downstream. This would infer a functional deficiency pertaining to B_{12}.

Organic acids give us an indirect window into different metabolic pathways and the specific nutrients it takes to run those pathways optimally. Methylmalonic acid, for example, could be a window into B_{12}. Or 8-hydroxy-2'-deoxyguanosine can give us a window into vitamin C or other antioxidants. Low organic acids can signify that the problem is more chronic, and the nutrient deficiencies are even more severe. Both high and low organic acids can be a problem, and doctors need to take the patient's clinical picture into account before making a recommendation.

Organic acid tests can give us a window into carbohydrate metabolism, fat metabolism, B vitamin levels, methylation, neurotransmitter function, detoxification, and gut bacteria imbalances, to name a few.

NutrEval Profile Testing

The NutrEval Profile test is a comprehensive nutritional evaluation that assesses a person's nutritional status by analyzing various biomarkers in blood and urine samples, which may include these:

- **Amino Acids:** This part of the test measures levels of essential and nonessential amino acids in the blood, providing insight into protein intake, digestion, and absorption, as well as potential imbalances or deficiencies that may impact overall health.

- **Fatty Acids:** The test evaluates levels of various fatty acids, including omega-3 and omega-6, to assess dietary fat intake and balance. This information can help identify imbalances that may contribute to inflammation or other health issues.

- **Antioxidant Status:** The test measures levels of specific antioxidants—such as coenzyme Q10, glutathione, and vitamin E—to assess the body's antioxidant capacity and identify potential deficiencies or imbalances.

- **Vitamin and Mineral Status:** The NutrEval test assesses levels of various vitamins and minerals, including B vitamins, vitamin D, and magnesium, to identify deficiencies or imbalances that may impact overall health and well-being.

- **Metabolic Markers:** The test evaluates specific markers of metabolism—such as homocysteine,

methylmalonic acid, and pyroglutamic acid—
which can provide insight into energy production,
detoxification processes, and other metabolic
pathways.

- **Organic Acids**: The test measures levels of various
  organic acids in urine, which can help identify
  imbalances or deficiencies in specific metabolic
  pathways, such as the citric acid cycle, neurotransmitter
  metabolism, or gut health.

- **Toxic Elements**: The test may also assess levels of toxic
  elements, such as heavy metals, to identify potential
  exposure risks and evaluate the body's detoxification
  capacity.

Metabolomix

The Metabolomix tests are designed to evaluate an individual's nutritional status and metabolic function. This test is
essentially an abbreviated version of the NutrEval and requires
only a blood prick that can be done at home instead of a blood
draw that requires a lab or phlebotomist like the NutrEval. The
Metabolomix looks at the following biomarkers:

- **Organic acids**: Metabolomix primarily focuses on
  measuring levels of organic acids in urine. These
  organic acids provide information about various
  metabolic pathways, including energy production,

neurotransmitter metabolism, detoxification processes, and gut health.

- **Amino acids:** Metabolomix also assesses levels of essential and nonessential amino acids in blood plasma, similar to NutrEval, to evaluate protein intake, digestion, and absorption.

- **Oxidative stress markers:** The test includes an assessment of specific markers of oxidative stress, such as lipid peroxides and glutathione, to evaluate the body's antioxidant capacity.

The NutrEval provides a more comprehensive analysis including fatty acids, vitamin and mineral status, and toxic elements, while the Metabolomix primarily focuses on organic acids, amino acids, and oxidative stress markers.

Thyroid Medication Options

Let's compare and contrast thyroid medications here. Most medications are going to be in the category of one the following:

- Natural desiccated thyroid (NDT) medication or over-the-counter supplement
- Natural compounded T4/T3 medication
- Synthetic thyroid hormone T4 or T3 thyroid hormone with a sodium salt attached to it

Liothyronine (T3) Sodium

$HO - \bigcirc - O - \bigcirc - CH_2 - C(NH_2)(H) - COO\,Na$

Levothyroxine (T4) Sodium

$HO - \bigcirc - O - \bigcirc - CH_2 - C(NH_2)(H) - COO\,Na \cdot xH_2O$

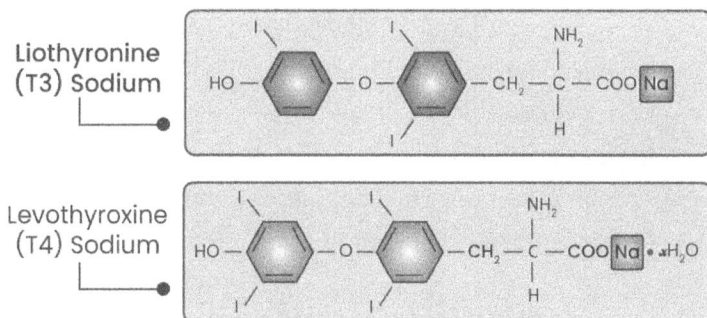

Conversion Chart

Here is an excellent conversion chart you can reference for better understanding of thyroid dosage equivalency among the different thyroid brands.

Nature-Thyroid (Thyroid USP)	WP-Thyroid (Thyroid USP)	Armour / NP Thyroid (Thyroid USP)	Synthetic T4 (Levothyroxine)	Synthetic T3 (Liothyronine)
1/4 grain (16.25mg)	1/4 grain (16.25mg)	1/4 grain (15 mg)	25 mcg	5 mcg
1/2 grain (32.5 mg)	1/2 grain (32.5 mg)	1/2 grain (30 mg)	50 mcg	
3/4 grain (48.75 mg)	3/4 grain (48.75 mg)		75 mcg	
			88 mcg	
1 grain (65 mg)	1 grain (65 mg)	1 grain (60 mg)	100 mcg	25 mcg
			112 mcg	
1.25 grain (81.25 mg)	1.25 grain (81.25 mg)		125 mcg	
			137 mcg	
1.5 grain (97.5 mg)	1.5 grain (97.5 mg)	1.5 grain (90 mg)	150 mcg	
1.75 grain (113.75 mg)	2 grain (130 mg)		175 mcg	
2 grain (130 mg)	1.75 grain (113.75 mg)	2 grain (120 mg)	200 mcg	50 mcg
2.25 grain (146.25 mg)				
2.5 grain (162.5 mg)				
3 grain (195 mg)		3 grain (180 mg)*	300 mcg	
4 grain (260 mg)		4 grain (240 mg)*		
5 grain (325 mg)		5 grain (300 mg)*		

1 grain = 38 mcg to T4 & 9 mcg T3

Source: United States Pharmacopeia—Drug Information 2000, 20th Edition
Armour® is a registered trademark of Allergan, Inc.
NP Thyroid® is a registered trademark of Acella, LLC.

T4-Only Medications

- Synthroid tablets
- Levoxyl tablets
- Levothyroxine generic
- Tirosint gel caps or Tirosint liquid (very clean; no fillers)
- Compounded T4 medications

T4/T3 Combination Medications

- WP Thyroid, Nature-Throid (Westhroid) (65 mg per grain, contains 38 mcg of T4 and 9 mcg of T3)
- Armour Thyroid or NP Thyroid (60 mg per grain, contains 38 mcg of T4,and 9 mcg of T3)
- Desiccated thyroid glandular (these tend to be over the counter)
- Compounded T4/T3 medications

Levothyroxine, a synthetic form of the thyroid hormone T4, is the second most prescribed drug in the United States and is widely used around the world. When a drug becomes generic, it loses its patent, allowing multiple pharmaceutical companies to produce their own versions of the medication. For example, levothyroxine is offered under various brand names by different manufacturers, including Synthroid®, Levothroid®, Levoxyl®, Unithroid®, and Thyro-Tabs®, primarily used in the United States. There are some cleaner forms of T4 without the fillers (I will elaborate more on this later), including Tirosint® liquid and gel versions. Other countries have different brands, including Eltroxin® (in Canada), Euthyrox® (in the EU), and Oroxine® or Eutroxsig® (in Australia).

T4-containing medications are typically initiated at a dose of 25 to 50 mcg per day (which is equivalent to one-fourth to one-half a grain of T4/T3 NDT glandular) and then gradually increased by 25 mcg per day every month or so, depending on the patient's thyroid lab results and symptoms. The typical maximum recommended dose is 300 mcg per day, or 3 grains of NDT. Starting low and slow and gradually increasing the dose can reduce side effects.

Levothyroxine or synthetic T4 medications are well established, typically well tolerated, and low cost due to their off-patent status. Most conventional doctors are familiar with and prescribe T4 medications due to their educational training and the influence of pharmaceutical companies. T4 medications have only been used since the 1970s, when they were first introduced by Merck. Before that, NDT glandular medications like Armour had been prescribed since the early 1900s. NDT thyroid glandulars are primarily porcine or pig derived, as pig glandular tissues seem to be more biocompatible with humans compared to bovine or cow thyroid tissue, for instance.[6]

Most conventional doctors prefer synthetic thyroid medications due to their standardized dosages, despite a possible 10 percent variation according to industry standards. In contrast, NDT glandular medications are USP certified, ensuring correct potency and amounts with an average 2 percent variation. Some doctors may not be aware of this and believe that NDT glandular medications have doses that vary significantly. If choosing over-the-counter NDT supplements, ensure the sources are reputable and confirm optimal thyroid levels through lab tests.

Over the last decade, there have been recalls on various thyroid medications due to doses exceeding the FDA's 10 percent acceptable range. This happened with synthetic T4 medications, including Levoxyl in 2014, Synthroid in 2013, and Tirosint in 2023.[7] This also happened on the natural side in 2020 with Nature-Throid (Westhroid) and WP Thyroid, which are all made by the same company, RLC Labs.[8] In 2023, the only NDT thyroid medications on the market are Armour and NP thyroid. Either way, it's always good to test your thyroid labs quarterly to ensure your levels are where they need to be. If, by chance, there is a thyroid dosing issue, you should be able to catch it early on and adjust your dose.

A drawback of many T4 medications, except for Tirosint and compounded T4, is the presence of fillers. Some of these fillers include calcium phosphate, colloidal silicon dioxide, corn starch, lactose, magnesium stearate, various dyes, acacia, confectioners' sugar (containing corn starch), lactose monohydrate, povidone (iodine), and talc.

While major drug companies may claim their medication is gluten-free, this often refers only to wheat, barley, and rye. For those sensitive to autoimmune triggers, corn and iodine could cause an immune system flare-up.

Other Ingredients in NDT Thyroid Glandulars

Brands to disclose:

- **WP Thyroid**: Inulin from chicory root, medium-chain triglycerides derived from coconut, lactose (added premanufacturing)[9]

- **Westhroid and Nature-Throid**: colloidal silicon dioxide, dicalcium phosphate, magnesium stearate, microcrystalline cellulose, croscarmellose sodium, stearic acid, Opadry II 85f19316 clear—tablet coating, lactose (added premanufacturing)

Brands that don't disclose:

- **NP Thyroid**: calcium stearate, dextrose monohydrate, maltodextrin (corn derived) and mineral oil[10]

- **Armour Thyroid**: Calcium stearate, dextrose, microcrystalline cellulose, sodium starch glycolate, Opadry white[11]

Side Note: All major thyroid glandular brands purchase their glandular tissue from the same supplier, American Laboratories, Inc. They add 5 mg of lactose per grain of thyroid tissue, which is 99.99 percent lower than the lactose that is in a glass of milk (13,000 mg) and should still be tolerated even if you are dairy or lactose intolerant.

The thyroid tissue is then sent out from American Laboratories to the pharmaceutical companies, where they manufacture the tissue into tablet forms. NP and Armour do not disclose the lactose in their glandular tissue, even though it is present premanufacturing. Therefore, the cleanest out of all the NDT glandulars is WP thyroid, based on their current ingredient list.

T3-Only Medications

- Liothyronine
- Cytomel
- Compounded T3 medications

Triiodothyronine (T3) is the primary thyroid hormone that is biologically active in our bodies. Although the thyroid gland secretes around 20 percent of T3 directly, the remaining 80 percent is produced through the natural conversion of thyroxine (T4) within our bodies. While both T4 and T3 have biological effects, T3 is three times more metabolically active than T4. It plays a critical role in ensuring that our bodies produce healthy levels of T3.

T3 is responsible for increasing metabolic rate, aiding in weight loss, and supporting energy production to keep us alert and stimulate the heart. Similar to T4, T3 can also lower TSH levels.

Some doctors prefer to use T3 alone due to difficulties in converting synthetic T4 to T3. However, in rare cases, patients taking NDT (natural desiccated thyroid) medications such as Nature-Throid may convert an excessive amount of T4 into RT3 (reverse T3). This excessive conversion can affect the ability of T3 to bind to its receptor sites. Nonetheless, such occurrences are uncommon but possible.

Some doctors rely only on T3 medications as they can lower TSH to a normal range. However, T4 does have a role in the body, helping to repair your brain, help with bone growth, and repair blood vessels. It is important you avoid T3-only medications unless you are testing to ensure you have adequate levels of T4 in your system as well. If you take NDT support, you will get both T4 and T3.

My general approach is to start with thyroid support in the following order:

1. Start with an NDT medication or supplement. This works 95 percent of the time.
2. If NDT is not tolerated, Tirosint T4 (no fillers) is your next step.
3. If T4 does not convert to T3 optimally, add in a T3-only medication till T3 is at optimal lab levels.
4. A compounded T4/T3 medication. I recommend this only if there is significant sensitivity with the NDT glandular resulting in an increase in thyroid antibodies and you also can't convert T4 to T3 adequately.

> **Important reminder**: It's important that all diet, lifestyle, and other thyroid-supporting nutrients are in place before adjusting your thyroid medications. When everything is in place nutritionally, I find less thyroid medication is needed.

What Should You Do If Your Thyroid Antibodies Increase?

Be careful not to hyper-fixate on every deviation your thyroid antibodies make. There is a natural day-to-day deviation of

TPO and thyroglobulin antibodies in general. Food plays a significant role, as do gut inflammation, gut permeability, nutrient deficiencies, infections, toxin exposure, and too much iodine. You need to ensure you are addressing the entire picture if you have elevated antibodies. Sometimes, as patients heal, their antibodies elevate as their immune system gets healthier, which needs to be considered as you move through your functional medicine program.

I have seen many patients test in the thousands regarding antibody elevation, and even some lower their antibodies below the lab threshold for testing positive. Some come and see me with much milder elevations as well. With some patients, it may not be possible to get their antibodies to test negative, but I routinely see a 50 percent reduction of thyroid antibodies (the same can be said for Graves' disease as well). I tell patients that an excellent goal to relieve Hashimoto's symptoms is to get their thyroid antibodies (TPO ab) below the 300 to 500 range.

I have seen patients with elevated TSI or TRAb on the Graves' hyperthyroid side, where previously those antibodies were causing excess T4 and T3 and very low TSH. We may see a gentle drop in TSI and TRAb, but those levels may still remain elevated, as they are not creating the elevated thyroid hormone levels or hyperthyroid symptoms they once did.

I always like to get an assessment of where someone's antibodies are at their worst and look for a minimum 50 percent drop. Some patients may get their antibodies tested for the first time after they have gotten much healthier regarding their diet, lifestyle, and gut health. We may not have an accurate indication of where their antibody starting point was. It was more than likely much higher, thus skewing what the overall anti-body reduction could have been.

Other Benefits of Natural Desiccated Thyroid

- **T2:** Another important thyroid hormone is T2, which is often overlooked. T2 is present only in NDT and plays a significant role in improving the body's ability to burn fat effectively by activating brown fat and increasing the body's metabolic rate. It also supports mitochondrial and ovarian function, as well as fertility. Like T4 and T3, T2 does affect TSH levels, which means if you are hypothyroid, adding in T2 directly or through an NDT could be advantageous based on my personal experience.

- **Calcitonin:** Calcitonin is a hormone responsible for regulating calcium and phosphate levels in the bloodstream. It achieves this by counteracting the impact of parathyroid hormone and ensuring that minerals remain at appropriate levels. Furthermore, calcitonin has a function in regulating the concentration of calcium and potassium in the body.

- **Protomorphogens (PMG):** Protomorphogens (PMG) are extracts derived from nucleic acids found in the cell nucleus and are present in glandular tissues. Many doctors have observed that when added to a patient's thyroid treatment regimen, PMG supplements enhance thyroid rebuilding and reduce thyroid antibodies, because these nucleic acids play a significant role in controlling the functions of the cell.

Thyroid Maintenance and Hormone Support

Thyroid maintenance should start with targeted lab work so you know what nutrients you need and what specific support you may need. Dialing in your diet is going to be foundational to ensuring you are getting healthy fats, proteins, and all of the nutrients you need for optimal thyroid function. An additional high-quality multivitamin and thyroid nutrients may be necessary to help your body synthesize thyroid hormone as well as activate and convert it. Your hormones function and dysfunction together, so looking at how your other hormone systems are doing (adrenals, thyroid, female, male, etc.) is important to help ensure optimal thyroid health.

If you would like my support in finding a qualified practitioner, I have a podcast available. The link is in the resources section. Look for "How to Find a Good Functional Medicine Practitioner."

Graves' Support

In Chapter 1, we briefly discussed Graves' disease. Here are some natural strategies that can help support Graves' disease. It is crucial to ensure that you are stable and are not experiencing severe thyroid storm symptoms like heart palpitations, high blood pressure, nausea, high pulse rate or excessively high thyroid hormone levels, as these can pose risks such as stroke. If you have time to incorporate natural strategies, the recommendations we provided in the book—including dietary adjustments, blood sugar management, infection support, gluten foundational nutrient support, sleep optimization, and lifestyle modifications—are all foundational to any other additional supplementation. With this solid foundation, my clinical experience is that any additional supplementation for hypothyroidism seems to work better and provide a greater clinical benefit. Please make sure you don't confuse Graves' disease and hyperthyroidism with Hashimoto's, as they can overlap, as I mentioned in earlier chapters. Many time patients with Graves' disease call also have Hashimoto's disease at the same time, so it's good to test for Hashimoto's antibodies as well as Graves' antibodies.

Additionally, working with a functional medicine doctor, you may consider incorporating specific nutrient support:

- **Carnitine**: L-Carnitine is an amino acid that may help reduce hyperthyroid symptoms by blocking the entry of excessive thyroid hormones into the cells. Typical dosage ranges from 1 to 5 g per day, but it should be used under the guidance of a health care professional.[12]

- **Selenium**: Selenium is a trace mineral that plays a role in thyroid hormone metabolism and may help regulate thyroid function. Dosage recommendations typically range from 200 to 400 mcg per day, but individual needs may vary.[13]

- **Lithium Orotate**: Lithium orotate is a mineral compound that has been suggested to help modulate thyroid function and reduce symptoms associated with Graves' disease. Dosage recommendations range from 5 to 10 mg per day, but it should be used under medical supervision.[14]

- **Lemon Balm:** Lemon balm (Melissa officinalis) is an herb known for its calming properties and may help alleviate anxiety and nervousness associated with Graves' disease. It can be consumed as a tea or taken in supplement form.[15]

- **Motherwort:** Motherwort (Leonurus cardiaca) is an herb that has been traditionally used to support cardiovascular health and reduce symptoms of hyperthyroidism. It may help calm heart palpitations and promote a sense of relaxation. It is usually taken as a tea or tincture.[16]

- **Bugleweed:** Bugleweed (Lycopus europaeus) is an herb that has been used to manage hyperthyroidism symptoms. It may help regulate thyroid hormone levels and reduce excessive thyroid activity. It is commonly taken as a tincture or tea.[17]

- **Higher dose iodine therapy:** Iodine therapy has been used in the past to stimulate a Wolff-Chaikoff effect, when the thyroid glands stop bringing iodine (more than 10 mg) into the thyroid, and thyroid hormone synthesis is temporarily halted for two to three weeks, creating a hypothyroid state. This type of therapy is one that you would try only while under the care of your functional medicine practitioner and endocrinologist.[18]

Nutritional Support for Other Body Systems

In addition to the thyroid, the body connections that help keep the thyroid balanced and functioning properly also need to be healthy. These include all of the systems covered in this book: the gut, the adrenals, the liver and detoxification, and the immune system.

There are many different options for supplemental support listed below. The goal isn't to take all of them, but to test and assess what may be the highest priority for your body.

Adrenal, Male and Female Support

Remember that the hormonal systems (thyroid, adrenals, male and female hormones) function and dysfunction together. A deficiency in one of them can create a chain reaction in the others. Some of the adaptogenic herbal support may be better for different adrenal patterns (high or low adrenal patterns), so there are different levels of individualizing a plan using the patient's clinical symptoms, history, and lab tests to make an optimal recommendation. You can at least get an idea of some of the adrenal nutrients and support that might be used below, but they are not limited to these:

- Vitamin C (ascorbic acid, l-ascorbate, buffered C, and with bioflavonoids are good)
- Vitamin B_1 (thiamine)
- Vitamin B_2 (riboflavin)
- Vitamin B_3 (niacin)
- Vitamin B_5 (pantothenic acid)
- Vitamin B_6 (as pyridoxal 5'-phosphate)

- B$_9$ (folate, calcium folinate, or L-5-MTHF)
- Vitamin B$_{12}$ (as methyl, adenosyl, or hydroxocobalamin)
- L-carnitine
- Eleuthero root (may require testing)
- American ginseng (may require testing)
- Ashwagandha root (may require testing)
- Rhodiola rosea (may require testing)
- Licorice (may require testing)

Additionally, the following supplements may be used for female or male hormone support:

- DHEA (requires testing—male and female)
- Pregnenolone (requires testing)
- Progesterone (requires testing)
- Estriol or estradiol (requires testing)
- Black cohosh extract
- Dong quai
- Chaste tree or vitex
- Maca
- Damiana
- Tribulus

Digestive Support

Remember that you need a healthy level of beneficial bacteria for a healthy gut and immune function. When there's an accompanying autoimmune condition, it's important to get the inflammation in the gut calmed down before we start clearing out the dysbiotic bad bacteria and then supporting the healthy beneficial bacteria.

There are many different supplements we can use for our digestive system. There is an ideal timing of when to use each supplement based on the 6R rule and taking the patient's labs, clinical symptoms, and history into account. Below are the supplements, but they are not limited to these:

- Probiotics (Lactobacillus, Bifidobacterium, Saccharomyces boulardii, bacillus and other spore-based organisms, Akkermansia)
- Betaine hydrochloride (HCl)
- Pepsin (enzyme)
- Amylase (enzyme for carbs)
- Protease (enzyme for proteins)
- Lipase (enzymes for fats)
- Ox bile (fat digestive support)
- Lactase (enzyme for dairy)
- DPP IV (enzymes for incidental gluten)

When the gut issues are addressed, so is the ability to absorb nutrients. The immune system is cooled down and the body can run its detoxification pathways much better.

Liver and Detox Support

When the liver works better, you are able to activate thyroid hormone better and convert T4 to T3—and 60 percent of that happens in the liver. There are many different supplements that can be used to support the liver and detoxification systems, and these include but are not limited to the following:

- Sulfur amino acids (glutamine, NAC or cysteine, glycine, taurine, leucine, methionine, MSM, ornithine)
- Milk thistle or silymarin
- Dandelion root
- Glutathione (reduced, liposomal or acetylated forms are good)
- Vitamin C (ascorbic acid, L-ascorbate, buffered c, and with bioflavonoids are good)
- Antioxidants (green tea, resveratrol, grape seed extract, curcumin, etc.)
- Calcium D-glucarate, DIM (Diindolylmethane)
- Selenium
- Molybdenum

Immune and Infection Support

Infections keep the gut and body inflamed, fuel autoimmunity, and prevent hormonal and other body systems from functioning optimally. There's a broad spectrum of supplements that can be used to eliminate infections. These were covered in "The Infection Connection" (Chapter 7), but to summarize here, they include the following:

- Samento
- Banderol
- Sida acuta
- Cryptolepis
- Reishi mushroom
- Cordyceps mushroom

- Echinacea
- Astragalus
- Elderberry
- Noni

- Vitamin D
- Vitamin A
- Neem

Additional Supplements to Consider

There are many additional supplements to consider, depending on your situation and your nutritional needs. I've summarized a few below. This is why it's helpful to work with someone to help prioritize and consolidate your specific supplement plan.

Protein Powder

Protein powders, including varieties such as pea-based, grass-fed collagen peptides, grass-fed whey, or grass-fed beef, boast impressive amino acid profiles. These profiles are rich in sulfur-containing amino acids, essential components that support the body in synthesizing glutathione. These protein powders can work as a meal replacement, and they can take stress off your digestion, which is perfect when you're in a hurry and trying to get healthy food into your body fast. A protein shake with amino acids and other nutrients in it can make a meal really easy for you. You could also mix in some dehydrated veggie greens, a handful of low-sugar fruit, or some coconut milk to craft a delicious and nutritious meal replacement.

Collagen is especially good as it's very high in the amino acid glycine, which is great for the lining, helps support healthy glutathione levels, and provides great building blocks for your connective tissues (cartilage, joints, skin, hair, and nails).

Resistant Starch

Resistant starches, such as cooled potato starch or unripened banana flour, can serve as an excellent supplement as they nourish beneficial gut bacteria. The microbes in the gut produce butyrate by fermenting dietary fibers. As a short-chain fatty acid, butyrate supplies energy to colon cells, reduces inflammation, and lowers the pH in the large intestine. This acidic environment makes it difficult for harmful, dysbiotic bacteria to thrive.

Resistant starches contribute to gut health by creating an environment that's slightly acidic, which discourages harmful bacteria from multiplying and encourages beneficial bacteria to flourish. This equilibrium is key because beneficial bacteria, such as *Lactobacillus acidophilus*—which means "acid-loving" in Latin—create important nutrients, while harmful bacteria can produce toxins. Therefore, incorporating resistant starches into your diet can improve the gut's microbial balance, lowering toxin levels and fostering a healthier probiotic population.

Colonics

Colonics might offer temporary relief, especially if you're dealing with constipation. However, they can't resolve infections or correct bacterial imbalances in your gut. While colonics can assist mechanically in moving stool through the colon, addressing the underlying causes of slow motility is crucial. These include issues like poor digestion, infections, and bacterial imbalances, which are often the reasons behind impaired stool movement. It's important to use colonics judiciously, as frequent use can disrupt electrolyte levels and the healthy bacterial balance in the colon.

Epsom Salt Baths

Magnesium can be taken orally, but with gut issues, it may be easier to absorb it via the skin, which can be a great way to relax at bedtime. Epsom salt can be great because you can get a very high amount of magnesium sulfate into your body through your skin without creating a laxative effect.

You can use a foot basin, which can be filled up to your ankles with hot water. An 8-ounce cup of Epsom salts can be added to the water to provide a sufficient dose. You can let your feet soak for about fifteen to twenty minutes, or until the water gets cold.

Chelation Therapy

Mercury and lead can aggravate thyroid autoimmune conditions. If there are high levels of lead or mercury, you may need to use chelation support (DMPS, DMSA, or EDTA) to help remove the metals. Along with chelation therapy, binders like citrus pectins, activated charcoal, chlorella, and bentonite clay can be used to bind up those metals to avoid recirculation. Amino acids (cysteine, glutamine, glycine, etc.) that increase glutathione as well as glutathione itself can be used to help up-regulate your cytochrome p450 oxidase Phase II pathways, which are needed for natural heavy metal detoxification.

Anytime you're dealing with chelation, you must work with a skilled functional medicine practitioner or a doctor to assure it is done safely. You also need to make sure chelation therapy is the last thing done in any program. You really want the gut to be working well before chelation is performed. Be very careful when using the chelation compounds via an IV, as the dose is much more potent and has the potential for serious side effects if not administered properly.

What to Look for in a Supplement

When purchasing supplements, look for high-quality supplements. Many use fillers such as gluten, which you want to avoid. In the world of supplements, you truly get what you pay for. Look for supplement companies that are recognized and do independent testing on their products.

Questions to which you will want to find answers include the following:

- Are fillers used, and if so, what kind?
- Are the supplements free from lead, molds, mycotoxins, and other chemicals?
- Do they buy from reputable supply chains? Price tends to factor in here.
- Are the supplements stored in a climate-controlled, low-humidity warehouse?
- Are high-quality ingredients used, such as folate instead of folic acid, or methyl B12 rather than cyanocobalamin? Are superior forms of magnesium used, like magnesium glycinate or magnesium malate, instead of magnesium oxide? And does it contain vitamin A directly, instead of relying on the less expensive precursor, beta-carotene?
- Are you getting mixed tocopherols for your vitamin E, or just the D-alpha tocopherol?

How to Find High-Quality Supplements

I get asked all the time what supplements I use. Check out the table below to get a sense of what those quality supplements are and what category they fall into. There are some great supplements out there, but I would say the majority are poor quality or potentially counterfeit. Be careful when procuring supplements from eBay and Amazon unless they are coming directly from the manufacturer or an authorized reseller, as there have been many reports of fraud and counterfeit products, as reported by the *New York Times* in 2015.[19]

This at least gives you an idea of what I use for myself and my patients. You can compare them against supplements you may already be taking. When purchasing products make sure they are from top-tier companies; typically these companies will charge more due to the high-quality raw ingredients, and their products are independently tested for potency without added excipients like mold and heavy metals, etc. Many have been around for decades and will have a reputation that exceeds them. Most will use an easy-to-break-down cellulose capsule so the supplements open and assimilate well, allowing for maximal absorption.

Flowing agents are used in some products like vegetable stearate, magnesium stearate, silicon dioxide, or silica, which are also safe and cause no concern. For instance, magnesium is an essential nutrient, and stearic acid is a saturated fat found in eggs, grass-fed beef, chicken, and nuts. These are used as flowing agents to ensure the nutrients are mixed well without clumping and allow for the supplement mixture to be homogenous with an equal amount of nutrients per capsule. Feel free to visit the resources section at the back of the book for additional guidance on the supplement topic.

Body System Categories	Supplements
Stomach Acid Support	Enzyme Synergy, HCL Supreme, Digest Synergy (lower dose HCL version if you are sensitive)
Liver and Detoxification Support	Antioxidant Supreme (Phase I detox), Detox Aminos (Phase II detox), Heavy Metal Clear, Liver Supreme
Thyroid Support	Thyro Balance, Thyro Replete, Iodine Synergy (lower dose iodine—make sure antibodies are stable before taking this)
Blood Sugar	Ashwagandha Supreme, Adrenal Revive, Emulsi D Supreme, Gluco Synergy
Nutrients	Amino Acid Supreme, CoQ10 Supreme, Curcumin Supreme, Iron Supreme, Magnesium Supreme, Multi Nutrient Supreme, TruCollagen (grass-fed)
Hormones	Cycle Balance (progesterone), Meno Balance (estriol), Femmenessence Cycling (maa specific to cycling), Femmenessence Meno (maca specific for menopause)
Adrenals	Adrenal Boost (glandular), Adrenal Revive, B-Vitamin Synergy, Licorice Drops, Mito Synergy, Pregnenolone Drops, and more!
Gut Support	HCL Supreme, Digest Synergy, Enzyme Synergy, GI Restore Powder, Megasporebiotic, Probio Flora, TruFiber (prebiotics)
GI Clearing	GI Clear 1, GI Clear 2, GI Clear 3, GI Clear 4, GI Clear 5, GI Clear 6

KEY POINTS

1. Make sure your nutrient levels are dialed in. Use a nutrient counter app to see if there are nutrients missing in your diet. Add supplements where you are having a hard time getting enough nutrients from food.

2. Some people need more nutrients, and getting high-quality nutrient tests like an organic acids test or an intracellular nutrient panel can help when making more specific supplement recommendations. See below for specific test options.

3. Nutrients like vitamin D may be difficult to get enough of from the sun alone, especially at higher latitudes, and where there's winter, supplementation is going to be essential.

4. If you have a known thyroid problem, look at the core thyroid nutrients for thyroid synthesis and conversion like selenium, magnesium, zinc, vitamin A, glutathione, and iodine (in small amounts if antibodies are stable).

5. Make sure you check with your allopathic doctor before you start natural Graves' or hyperthyroid support.

6. If you are having any digestive issues, make sure you are digesting your food well. Using HCL, enzymes, and/or bile salts can help ensure you are breaking down and absorbing the nutrients from your food.

Resources

Thyroid Reboot Foundations Bundle (www.justinhealth. com/foundations) Here are several recommended thyroid-supporting supplements mentioned in the book in easy-to-access bundles.

Just In Health Supplements (www.justinhealth.com/shop) You can find various supplements that I use personally as well as recommend to my patients. They are organized by categories for easy browsing.

Micronutrients Counter (www.justinhealth.com/nutrient-counter) This is a nutrient counter that will track your macronutrients like protein, fat, carbs, and overall calories, which is standard for an app like this. What's different about this one is that it will also look at micronutrients like magnesium, potassium, etc.

Organic Acid Test OAT (www.justinhealth.com/organic-acid-test) This test looks at organic acids, giving us a window into the function of metabolic processes in the body like detoxification, mitochondrial function, nutritional deficiencies, gut bacteria, and fungal overgrowth.

Blood Test Review (www.justinhealth.com/blood-test-road-map) This is an Excel sheet that contains the reference range for thyroid labs as well as other tests I use.

Urinary Iodine Test (www.justinhealth.com/iodine-test) This is a twenty-four-hour urinary test to assess iodine levels.

NutrEval Test (www.justinhealth.com/nutreval-test) This is a comprehensive analysis that identifies nutritional deficiencies and imbalances in the body. By examining various biomarkers, it provides insights into one's metabolic health, including amino acid, fatty acid, and antioxidant levels.

MetabolomiX+ Test (www.justinhealth.com/metabolimx-test) This is a comprehensive assessment that evaluates an individual's metabolic health and function. By analyzing blood and urine, it provides insights into one's nutritional status, energy production, and detoxification processes.

Micronutrients Deficiency Test (www.justinhealth.com/micronutrient-deficiency-test) This test is an advanced diagnostic tool that uses lymphocyte stimulation to assess micronutrient levels and cellular function in the body. By evaluating vitamins, minerals, antioxidants, and other essential nutrients, it identifies deficiencies and imbalances.

Notes

1   Leonidas H. Duntas, "Nutrition and Thyroid Disease," *Current Opinion in Endocrinology, Diabetes and Obesity* 30, no. 6 (December 2023): 324–29, https://doi.org/10.1097/MED.0000000000000831.

2   Zimmermann and Köhrle, "The Impact of Iron and Selenium Deficiencies on Iodine and Thyroid Metabolism."

3   Morelly L. Maayan, Rocco V. Sellitto, and Eugene M. Volpert,
     "Dopamine and L-Dopa: Inhibition of Thyrotropin-Stimulated
     Thyroidal Thyroxine Release," *Endocrinology* 118, no. 2 (February
     1, 1986): 632–36, https://doi.org/10.1210/endo-118-2-632; and J. R.
     Strawn et al., "Pituitary-Thyroid State Correlates with Central
     Dopaminergic and Serotonergic Activity in Healthy Humans,"
     Neuropsychobiology 49, no. 2 (February 2004): 84–87, https://doi.
     org/10.1159/000076415.

4   Zimmermann and Köhrle, "The Impact of Iron and Selenium
     Deficiencies on Iodine and Thyroid Metabolism."

5   Koji Aoyama, "Glutathione in the Brain," *International Journal of
     Molecular Sciences* 22, no. 9 (2021): 5010, https://doi.org/10.3390/
     ijms22095010.

6   Elizabeth A. McAninch and Antonio C. Bianco, "The History
     and Future of Treatment of Hypothyroidism," *Annals of Internal
     Medicine* 164, no. 1 (2016): 50–56, https://doi.org/10.7326/M15-1799.

7   "RLC Labs, Inc., Issues Voluntary Nationwide Recall of All Lots
     of Nature-Throid® and WP Thyroid® with current Expiry Due
     to Sub Potency," Food and Drug Administration, September 3,
     2020, https://www.fda.gov/safety/recalls-market-withdrawals-
     safety-alerts/rlc-labs-inc-issues-voluntary-nationwide-
     recall-all-lots-nature-throidr-and-wp-thyroidr-current; Eric
     Palmer, "New Manufacturing Issues Lead AbbVie to 2nd
     Synthroid Recall," Fierce Pharma, January 14, 2013, https://
     www.fiercepharma.com/supply-chain/new-manufacturing-
     issues-lead-abbvie-to-2nd-synthroid-recall; and "Recall of
     TIROSINT® SOL (Levothyroxine Sodium) Oral Solution," Horizon
     NJ Health, accessed May 1, 2024, https://www.horizonnjhealth.
     com/membersupport/updates-and-announcements/
     recall-tirosint-sol-levothyroxine-sodium-oral-solution.

8   "Nature-Throid® (Thyroid USP) Tablets," RLC Labs, accessed May
     1, 2024, https://getrealthyroid.com/assets/docs/Nature-Throid-
     Prescribing-Information.pdf.

9   "WP Thyroid® (Thyroid USP) Tablets," RLC Labs, accessed May
     1, 2024, https://getrealthyroid.com/assets/docs/WP-Thyroid-
     Prescribing-Information.pdf.

10   "NP THYROID 60- Levothyroxine, Liothyronine Tablet," Acella
     Pharmaceuticals, LLC, last modified April 2023, https://dailymed.

nlm.nih.gov/dailymed/getFile.cfm?setid=f347f490-7199-4de6-bca2-0d44a74979af&type=pdf#:~:text=They%20contain%20both%20tetraiodothyronine%20sodium,(agglomerated)%20and%20mineral%20oil.

11   "Armour-Thyroid: Thyroid, Porcine Tablet," DailyMed, National Institutes of Health, last modified March 7, 2024, https://dailymed.nlm.nih.gov/dailymed/drugInfo.cfm?setid=56b41079-60db-4256-9695-202b3a65d13d.

12   Salvatore Benvenga et al., "Usefulness of L-Carnitine, a Naturally Occurring Peripheral Antagonist of Thyroid Hormone Action, in Iatrogenic Hyperthyroidism: A Randomized, Double-Blind, Placebo-Controlled Clinical Trial," *Journal of Clinical Endocrinology & Metabolism* 86, no. 8 (August 1, 2001): 3579–94, https://doi.org/10.1210/jcem.86.8.7747.

13   Konstantinos A. Toulis et al., "Selenium Supplementation in the Treatment of Hashimoto's Thyroiditis: A Systematic Review and a Meta-Analysis," *Thyroid* 20, no. 10 (October 2010): 1163–73, https://doi.org/10.1089/thy.2009.0351. This study highlights the role of selenium in autoimmune thyroid conditions.

14   Karin Broberg et al., "Lithium in Drinking Water and Thyroid Function," *Environmental Health Perspectives* 119, no. 6 (January 20, 2011): 827–30, https://doi.org/10.1289/ehp.1002678.

15   Daniel Kaplan and Chrysoula Dosiou, "Two Cases of Graves' Hyperthyroidism Treated with Homeopathic Remedies Containing Herbal Extracts from *Lycopus spp.* and *Melissa officinalis*," *Journal of the Endocrine Society* 5, suppl. 1 (April–May 2021): A971, https://doi.org/10.1210/jendso/bvab048.1984.

16   Radu Claudia Fierascu et al., "*Leonurus cardiaca* L. as a Source of Bioactive Compounds: An Update of the European Medicines Agency Assessment Report (2010)," *BioMed Research International* 2019 (April 17, 2019): 4303215, https://doi.org/10.1155/2019/4303215.

17   Kaplan and Dosiou, "Two Cases of Graves' Hyperthyroidism."

18   K. Markou et al., "Iodine-Induced Hypothyroidism," *Thyroid* 11, no. 5 (May 2001): 501–510, https://doi.org/10.1089/105072501300176462.

19   Anahad O'Connor, "New York Attorney General Targets Supplements at Major Retailers" *New York Times*, February 3, 2015, https://archive.nytimes.com/well.blogs.nytimes.com/2015/02/03/new-york-attorney-general-targets-supplements-at-major-retailers.

9

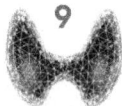

Connecting
It All Together

N THIS CHAPTER, WE WILL FOCUS ON CONNECTING all the important information from previous chapters, including the key takeaways. In the world of functional medicine, you do not want to wait until things get bad—until you are so unhealthy, sick, injured, or have hit rock bottom—before you get help. This is a stark contrast to the world of conventional medicine, where the expectation is that you will wait until you are sick or injured and then seek a doctor's help.

There were recently plumbers at my house doing some work on a leaky faucet. The next day, one plumber was looking for the leak but couldn't find it. He told his partner, "Well, maybe it just went away."

His partner stated, "Leaks never resolve by themselves. If there's a leak, it's only going to worsen." Then he increased the flow, inspected more thoroughly, and discovered the leak. The issue was that the plumbing system hadn't been under enough stress to make the leak obvious. The point is that problems like these don't just disappear. Similarly, with your body, the longer stress remains unaddressed in the background, the more pronounced the symptoms in your life become.

If you have low thyroid symptoms mentioned in the book—including fatigue, brain fog, hair loss, and weight gain, to name only a few—unfortunately, they will worsen if the root cause continues to be ignored. Do you want to wait until you are really sick and damage to your thyroid continues to accumulate? Or do you want to address the root causes of stress now?

I like to use the acronym PAIN, which means **p**ay **a**ttention **i**nside **n**ow. That's what we're telling you to do—pay attention inside now—whether it's aesthetic, inflammatory, mood, energy, or something else. Don't keep ignoring these symptoms until you hit rock bottom. The body is amazingly resilient, and as we start to take the stress out of your stress bucket, healing can start all on its own.

Connecting the Systems

The template for how functional medicine practitioners treat patients is pretty unique. It involves making connections between systems. Nutritionists will primarily focus on the diet part. Medical doctors often skip the diet and sometimes focus on hormones but ignore the gut. Other providers may work only on infections, such as Lyme disease, mold, or gut infections.

How do functional medicine practitioners excel as general practitioners, adept at identifying key issues across infections, hormones, diet, lifestyle, and the digestive system, and then integrate treatments to address all these areas simultaneously?

Moreover, how do they achieve this holistically, targeting the root cause unique to each individual? The root causes vary significantly from person to person; for example, one individual's health concerns might be 60 percent diet-related, 30 percent due to infections, and 10 percent hormone-related, while another's could be 30 percent diet, 50 percent hormones, and 20 percent gut-related.

Our approach involves assessing the most significant factors for each individual, understanding that these factors differ widely. Prioritizing these issues allows us to effectively address each one, maximizing the chances of resolving the core problems. In this final chapter, we aim to connect all three systems: diet and lifestyle, infections, and detoxification.

Diet and Lifestyle

Everything sits on a foundation, and the introductory foundation is diet and lifestyle. This includes the following:

- What you eat
- When you eat
- The quality of food that you eat
- How you sleep

- How you move
- How you deal with stress
- What you drink

Diet and lifestyle can look different depending on your level of health. The sicker you are, the more extreme the diet should be, as long as you can execute and follow through with it. The more drastic the initial changes, the faster the results will come.

Your diet must be dialed in specifically for you. If you're just a little bit unhealthy or sick, maybe you're kind of in the middle; that's not too bad. A Paleo template where there is nutritional density, foods are anti-inflammatory, and are low toxin may be a good starting point.

To briefly review, this means no grains, no legumes, and no dairy. If you've been unhealthy or sick for longer periods of time—maybe you have a history of autoimmunity in the family, have been diagnosed with autoimmunity yourself, or have autoimmune symptoms—the next step may be an autoimmune Paleo template. This is where we would go to the next step, which cuts out nuts, nightshades, and eggs.

From there, if you have excessive gut issues, there are special diets we may recommend. The specific carbohydrate diet (SCD) could help. It eliminates salicylates, phenols, and other anti-nutrients that could prevent the gut from healing. On this diet, all vegetables are peeled, everything is well cooked, and foods are mashed. A Gut and Psychology Syndrome (GAPS) approach may also be considered. This is where the focus is more on bone broth and soups.

Sometimes a low-FODMAP diet is used. This is a diet that cuts out fermentable oligosaccharides, disaccharides, mono-saccharides, and polyols, which are fermentable carbohydrates and fermentable sugars. It's possible that the low-FODMAP diet is added to or overlaps with any of the previous diets recommended. When this is added, it's done with the goal of starving out the dysbiotic bacteria in the gut and making it easier for your gut to digest food. Other goals include the avoidance of toxins from pesticides and chemicals (going organic can help here) and blood sugar stabilization.

It's also important that you aren't skipping meals and that you're getting good sleep. Water taken in between meals or ten minutes before meals is another strategy that should be included so you don't dilute digestive juices (enzymes and hydrochloric acid).

Gluten Recap

Going truly gluten free, covered in Chapter 5, means cutting out all grains and potential cross-reactive proteins like prol-amin. Even if you are one of the rare 10 percent who doesn't carry the gene for gluten sensitivity, gluten can still be inflam-matory and potentially impair mineral and protein absorption. However, once you have your health in check, if you don't have an active autoimmune condition or gluten sensitivity and your system can tolerate some grains and gluten, there are good, better, and best options.

Of course, the best option is to abstain from grains and glu-ten. If you need a cheat moment, the better grain option for most people tends to be white rice or even safer starches, such as yucca, plantains, sweet potatoes, and squash. If you feel that you can't entirely eliminate bread, a good option is sourdough, which is shown to have less gluten due to the fermentation process and easier to digest. The gliadin protein in gluten is broken down by lactic acid during the fermentation process, but not all the way. Sourdough would be the lesser of all the gluten evils when it comes to bread.

Emotional Stress

Another key building block in your foundation is neutralizing and eliminating emotional stress. If you are experiencing a lot of emotional stress due to ongoing issues—maybe you're in the middle of a divorce, there's been a death in the family, or there is work stress—this needs to be addressed. Not processing your emotional stress can negate your body's ability to heal. Remember that emotional stress is one of the three key stressors (emotional, physical, and chemical) that must be addressed in the Triangle of Health. Once you have recognized your emotional stressors, you can strategize ways to address them. Unresolved stress may decrease and even prevent your ability to heal. Even small action steps can relieve the anxiety caused by not doing anything in the first place. If you are going through significant emotional stress and you don't quite have your arms around it yet, you may need to adjust your healing goals until you do.

Infections

In your gut, there are good bacteria and bad bacteria that, if out of balance, could impact the immune system, making you more susceptible to infections. By weeding out the bad and nourishing the gut, it starts to put you on the healing path. To go through the complete process of healing, follow each step of the 6R strategy in the right order of priority:

1. **Remove** hyperallergenic foods (such as gluten)
2. **Replace** enzymes, acids, and bile salts
3. **Repair** with healing nutrients and adrenal support
4. **Remove** infections
5. **Reinoculate** with probiotics and prebiotics
6. **Retest** to assure infection is cleared

Here's a synopsis of these different steps:

1. Remove Hyperallergenic Foods (Such as Gluten)

This is covered in depth in the "Diet and Lifestyle" section earlier in this chapter, but simply put, it's about making sure you eat nutrient-dense, anti-inflammatory, low-toxin foods and eliminating those foods your body is sensitive to.

2. Replace Enzymes, Acids, and Bile Salt

Reflux, bloating, vertical ridging in the nails, undigested food, gray or floating stool, poor hair, or very dry skin are all symptoms that food is not digested optimally. To support the diet piece of the puzzle, digestive support should be brought to the forefront. You may use hydrochloric acid, enzymes, and/or bitters to help stimulate digestion. Without proper digestion, toxins build up in the system and negate the whole process of health, so addressing digestion early on is important. We may also focus on enhancing motility if constipation is still present even after diet and digestive support are added. We typically use nonabrasive nutrients like oxygenated magnesium and Triphala (which is a fruit) if needed.

3. Repair with Healing Nutrients and Adrenal Support

Supporting your adrenals and hormones can help reduce gut inflammation, heal the adrenals, and improve IgA levels, which are the localized immune system in the digestive tract. Healing nutrients are necessary for people who have extra gut inflammation or irritation. Things like L-glutamine, licorice root, deglycyrrhized licorice root, slippery elm, cat's claw, and amino acids (e.g., L-glutamine, Jerusalem artichoke, etc.)— these are healing nutrients that support the gut lining.

4. Remove Infections

Infections can be eliminated because of the three prior phases: removing the hyperallergenic foods; replacing the enzymes, acids, and bile salts; and repairing the gut lining and healing the adrenals with nutrients. After all these steps, you can start working on removing infections. The infections are determined by a stool test, which may test positive for H. pylori or a fungal or parasitic infection. The stool test may be positive for a variety of infections. Whatever the case, the infections need to be specifically addressed with unique protocols for each infection.

5. Reinoculate with Probiotics and Prebiotics

Once all the bad bacteria are weeded out of the gut, the reinoculation of the gut with probiotics reseeds the gut with good, healthy bacteria. Add in prebiotic fibers that act like fertilizer to help the good bacteria grow and gain a foothold in the microbiome.

Probiotics may also be added in the repair phase (step 3) because probiotics can have an anti-inflammatory effect and can help with motility. This type of recommendation is a deviation from the typical 6R strategy, but it may be necessary at times.

6. Retest to Assure Infections Are Cleared

Retesting for infections gives you the confidence and sense of completion that an important step in the progress has been made. It's also good to ensure that there are no hidden infections that burrowed deeper into the gut lining and could make their way to the surface or get reinfected from a spouse, partner, or family member.

Herbs versus Antibiotics Recap

In functional medicine, the conservative approach to taking care of your health and nurturing your body is the path to health. Part of this approach is the use of antimicrobial herbal medicines that have been around for literally thousands of years and have a strong safety profile. The types of herbal antimicrobials we use tend to be more selective for bad bacteria and less selective for good bacteria. There are many other benefits, including the targeting of efflux pumps, which antibiotics tend to miss.

Antibiotics, such as clarithromycin and amoxicillin, which may be prescribed for an H. pylori infection, may not work close to 30 percent of the time or more.[1] How many times have you been given an antibiotic prescription that just didn't completely clear up your infection? Your doctor likely prescribed an even stronger antibiotic to try again, which knocks down the remaining good bacteria as well. The overuse of antibiotics can also create more resistant strains, requiring tougher and stronger antibiotics the next time. Then when you really need an antibiotic for a serious infection, like a car accident that fractures your arm, the antibiotics may not work due to microbial resistance.

A 2016 study ranked medical error as the third-leading cause of death in the United States with 250,000 deaths per year.[2] In 2000, in the *Journal of the American Medical Association*, Barbara Starfield reported about the deficiencies in the US health care system.[3] At that time, there were seven thousand deaths per year due to hospital medication errors. This doesn't take into account any deaths due to prescribed and over-the-counter medications, including ibuprofen, which carries warnings of death due to heart failure and GI bleeding. The *New England Journal of Medicine* reports more than 16,500 deaths from NSAIDS among arthritis patients alone each year. You can imagine if you factor in all regular NSAID users, the number of deaths is much higher.[4] There are serious risks associated with the use of conventional medication.

Antibiotics can also create oxidative stress and mitochondrial dysfunction. The mitochondria are the powerhouse of the

CONNECTING IT ALL TOGETHER · 313

cell. They help generate ATP, which is an important raw material or source of energy in the body. Antibiotics also create oxidative stress, which is a way of breaking down the body. If you cut an apple open and leave it on the counter, it will turn brown due to oxidation. This internal oxidation creates a depletion of your antioxidant reserves. Then your body uses up more vitamin C, vitamin E, and other nutrients that would typically be used for other organ functions. And if you were to add some vitamin C from a fresh-cut lemon to that apple, the vitamin C would protect the apple from oxidizing and turning brown.

Antibiotics can cause oxidative stress and mitochondrial dysfunction as side effects. If you must use them, it's wise to explore gentler, natural alternatives before resorting to these stronger medications.

I've observed that patients on antibiotics often experience adverse effects, a scenario less common with antimicrobial herbs, partly due to the way these herbs kill and eliminate pathogens. I'm not entirely against antibiotics; in certain cases, they are necessary and effective. However, our preferred approach begins with herbs (step 1), followed by using synergistic herbs to minimize resistance (step 2). Only at step 3 do we consider antibiotics, complemented by herbal treatments and biofilm support, depending on the patient's progress and overall improvement in health.

Detoxification

Certain nutrients are required in the detoxification process. By eating nutritionally poor and toxic foods, your detoxification process will be suboptimal. By addressing system one—diet and lifestyle—right off the bat, you are already starting to work on detoxifying indirectly.

Do you recall the Phase I and Phase II detoxification processes we discussed in Chapter 7? In Phase I, we consume nutrient-rich foods that are then broken down into very fine particles, similar to how a garbage disposal works. Proteins are dismantled into their amino acid components, with sulfur-based amino acids playing a crucial role in Phase II. During Phase II, the detoxification process involves eliminating all the substances broken down in Phase I. This elimination occurs through the bile, stool, and kidneys, effectively flushing these compounds out of the body.

These metabolic reactions for detoxification include acetylation, hydroxylation, glutathione production, and methylation. Nutrients such as cysteine, glutamine, glycine, and taurine are needed for these processes to occur. If protein cannot be broken down into those smaller amino acids, Phase II will not occur optimally.

In cases of small intestinal bacterial overgrowth (SIBO), also known as dysbiosis, the natural production of healthy bacteria in the gut is suppressed. These beneficial bacteria are crucial because they generate a wealth of nutrients. Essentially, good bacteria consume waste and excrete valuable substances, like B vitamins and antioxidants. On the other hand, harmful bacteria consume these nutrients and excrete waste. An excess of harmful bacteria can increase toxicity in your body and burden your immune system.

Leaky Gut Recap

Remember, a leaky gut happens when those tight junctions become more permeable, allowing toxic gut particles to leak into the bloodstream. They recirculate back through the system. Leaky gut is really the consequence of all the inflammation in the gut. This inflammation accumulates from many sources, including food allergens, inadequate food breakdown, slow motility, infection, and bacterial imbalances. Leaky gut isn't necessarily the cause; it's more of an end result. To get your detoxification back on track, your digestive tract needs to be dialed in.

Detoxification Testing Recap

An organic acid test is typically a good starting point because it offers a window into various detoxification pathways. Whether it's pyroglutamate or other types of organic acids, the test will give us another window into how those sulfur aminos are doing.

Is the demand for the organic acids high, or are they depleted? You also get a window into B vitamin status, methylation, and oxidative stress by looking at 8-hydroxy-2'-deoxyguanosine. There are markers for the brain, the gut, and so on.

We may even look at tests like the micronutrient testing, organic acids (OAT), or urinary mold and toxin testing. The NutrEval metabolomics test is a hybrid between an organic acid urine test and an intracellular nutrient blood test. It gives us a good window into what's happening. We may run a heavy-metal challenge test with a chelation compound, like DMPS, DMSA, or EDTA. The chelation compound shows us what's

coming out in the urine, and a lot of times we can see aluminum, arsenic, cadmium, mercury, and lead.

If I discover on an organics test, for example, that a patient
has an increase in oxidative stress, I may add some extra vitamin C as part of the adrenal protocol. We have to make adjustments depending on the patient's needs.

You may be thinking, *Well, Dr. J gave me some detox support
while addressing Body System 1.* System 1 has to do with the
hormones (adrenal, thyroid, and female/male hormones). This
would have been dependent upon how you were presenting
(your symptoms), how sensitive you were, and how poor your
detoxification pathway was. Supplements may be added for
System 1. This could happen because the patient is overly sensitive due to poor detoxification and an up-regulated immune
system. Detoxification support may be necessary earlier in the
process to help lessen this sensitivity and allow the patient to
tolerate their adrenal support. This is why it's important to look
at each patient as an individual and meet them exactly where
they are on their journey.

Managing Your Lab Test Data—
Assessing, Not Guessing

In this book, we talked about many different functional lab
tests that you can run to assess how well or healthy your body
is—everything from blood tests, hormone tests, gut tests, infection tests, and heavy-metal and toxin-related tests. The more
data you gather, the more overwhelming it can be to chart and
keep track of it all. I dealt with many new patients coming in

with hundreds of pages of lab tests spanning over a decade. As a doctor, it becomes very overwhelming to look at this data and make heads or tails of it.

There is cutting-edge health-tracking software that has been developed to address this exact issue. This software allows you to graph all of your old data, making it easy to compare your old lab results with your new lab results. It can connect to wearables like your Fitbit, continuous glucose monitor (CGM), Oura ring, Apple Watch, etc. There's also a transcription service where you can upload all of your old lab PDFs, and a data-entry person will plug all that data in for you.

If you can measure it, you can improve it. Tracking your data will give you confidence that you are moving in the right direction.

Wrapping Things Up

There's a lot of information in this book, so it's very easy to feel overwhelmed and not quite sure where to start, and that's OK! Using the Japanese principle of *Kaizen*, which is the process of continually improving with small steps, is the easiest way to avoid feeling overwhelmed and to get the momentum you need from taking action, completing a task, and succeeding.

An easy, simple action, for example, could be just focusing on drinking clean, filtered mineral water as your primary source of hydration. Next could be a simple food change, like cutting out grains. The next change could be consuming a palm-sized amount of protein at each meal to help with blood sugar stability. You can continue to build on each recommendation with bigger or smaller bite-size tasks based on how well you feel.

The little dopamine hit you get from completing the tasks above will help propel you into the next day, feeling optimistic about the next new habit you are about to add. Just remember, if you fall off the horse, so to speak, that is OK. You are only one decision away from getting back on. Just brush yourself off and get back on!

Once we have grabbed all the low-hanging fruit of diet, lifestyle, and foundational supplement advice, the next step will be getting labs completed so we can look under the hood, so we are no longer guessing but assessing. If you get overwhelmed at all in this journey, you can see the resource section at the end of the book to help provide you with the support you need when you are ready.

KEY POINTS

1. The key takeaway from this book is that you do not want to wait until things get bad before you get help.

2. Your diet and lifestyle are foundational. In order for this to be effective, you must dial them both in. Utilize the free information here to build up your foundation.

3. Wiping out infections is system two, and this includes the 6R strategy shared many times throughout this book:
   a. Remove hyperallergenic foods
   b. Replace enzymes, acids, and bile salts

    c. Repair with healing nutrients and adrenal support

    d. Remove infections

    e. Reinoculate with probiotics and prebiotics

    f. Retest to assure infections are cleared

4. Detoxification is system three, and it's important to finish with detox, not start with it.

5. As Dr. Martin Luther King, Jr. said, remember: "Take the first step in faith. You don't have to see the whole staircase; just take the first step." I love this quote as I find many patients make things way bigger in their heads and psych themselves out from taking action.

6. As Dale Carnegie said, "Knowledge isn't power until it is applied." Make sure you apply at least one piece of information in this book and build on a new action every day or week. These slow and steady changes will eventually be locked into longer-lasting health habits over time.

7. Start with simple actions that you are confident you can follow through with. Feel the success of starting and completing a task. As your confidence improves, just add one more task at a time.

Resources

Access to Dr. J (www.justinhealth.com/free-consult) Here you can find virtual options to work with me if you want to dive in as a patient and get to the root of your thyroid and other health challenges.

Thyroid Reboot Foundations Bundle (www.justinhealth. com/foundations) Here are several recommended thyroid-supporting supplements mentioned in the book in easy-to-access bundles.

Access to The Thyroid Course (www.justinhealth.com/ thyroid-course) Here you can find my course, which is an in-depth video version of this course in a live lecture format. There are live Q & As to enhance your experience of the book.

Putting It Together (www.justinhealth.com/putting-it-together) Here is information on how to put together an optimal functional medicine program. It's important to address foundational issues while testing for root causes and stressors that are holding back your healing. This podcast will walk you through the right steps.

Find a Good Practitioner (www.justinhealth.com/find-a-practitioner) This podcast episode will explain how to find a practitioner who has a comprehensive approach, addresses the root causes of health issues, and offers personalized treatment plans. Consider compatibility in terms of communication and rapport, ensuring a strong patient–practitioner relationship for optimal health outcomes.

Health Tracker (www.justinhealth.com/health-tracker) Here you can efficiently manage and track your previous lab work.

Thyroid Reboot Recipes (www.justinhealth.com/thyroid-reboot-recipes) Dr. J's Thyroid Reboot Recipes will provide additional dietary advice and recipes to help supplement optimal thyroid health.

Notes

1   Yuhong Yuan et al., "Optimum Duration of Regimens for *Helicobacter pylori* Eradication," *Cochrane Database of Systematic Reviews*, no. 12 (December 11, 2013), https://doi.org/10.1002/14651858.CD008337.pub2.

2   Martin A. Makary and Michael Daniel, ""Medical Error—the Third Leading Cause of Death in the US,"" *BMJ* 353 (2016): i2139, https://doi.org/10.1136/bmj.i2139.

3   Barbara Starfield, "Is US Health Really the Best in the World?," *Journal of the American Medical Association* 284, no. 4 (2000): 483–85, https://doi.org/10.1001/jama.284.4.483.

4   ""Gastrointestinal Toxicity of Nonsteroidal Antiinflammatory Drugs,"" *New England Journal of Medicine* 341, no. 18 (October 28, 1999): 1397–99, https://doi.org/10.1056/NEJM199910283411813; and M. Michael Wolfe, David R. Lichtenstein, and Gurkirpal Singh, ""Gastrointestinal Toxicity of Nonsteroidal Antiinflammatory Drugs,"" *New England Journal of Medicine* 340, no. 24 (June 17, 1999): 1888–99, https://doi.org/10.1056/NEJM199906173402407.

Resources

I provide virtual health consultations and support worldwide, and you can reach me directly at www.justinhealth.com to schedule a consultation.

There will also be online courses available to the general public as well as to health providers that will act as a supplement to this book, *The Thyroid Reboot*. Access these here: www.justin health.com/thyroid-course. This is great for individuals and practitioners who want even more information and support.

Chapter 1

Access to Dr. J (www.justinhealth.com/free-consult) Here you can find virtual options to work with Dr. J if you want to dive in as a patient and get to the root of your thyroid and other health challenges.

Thyroid Reboot Foundations Bundle (www.justinhealth. com/foundations) Here are several of the recommended thyroid supporting supplements mentioned in the book in easy-to-access bundles.

Access to The Thyroid Course (www.justinhealth.com/thyroid-course) Here you can find Dr. J's course, which is an in-depth video version of this course in a live lecture format. There will be live Q&As to enhance your experience of the book.

Basal Temperature Instructions (www.justinhealth.com/temperature-test) This is an easy handout to chart your basal body temperature and assess your metabolism.

Blood Test Review (www.justinhealth.com/blood-test-road-map) This is an Excel sheet that contains the reference range for thyroid labs as well as other blood tests Dr. J uses.

Complete Thyroid Test (www.justinhealth.com/complete-thyroid-test) This is a comprehensive thyroid panel, including TSH, T4 free, T4 total, T3 free, T3 total, TPO ab, TG ab, and RT3.

Abridged Thyroid Test (www.justinhealth.com/abridged-thyroid-test) This is an abridged thyroid panel including TSH, T4 free, T3 free, TPO ab, and TG ab.

Thyroid Laser (www.justinhealth.com/thyroid-laser) Here you will be able to get information on purchasing or renting a therapeutic grade laser to help with thyroid inflammation and stimulate thyroid tissue healing.

Chapter 2

Thyroid Reboot Foundations Bundle (www.justinhealth.com/foundations) Here are several recommended thyroid supporting supplements mentioned in the book in easy-to-access bundles.

Meal Map Diet Handout (www.justinhealth.com/meal-map)
This is the quick-start diet guide that Dr. J used with
his patients. There are some simple diet and lifestyle
strategies laid out that are easy to follow.

Whole House Filtration (www.justinhealth.com/water-filters)
This is a recommendation for the whole-house filter Dr. J
uses in his own home. This filter is carbon-based and has a
pre- and post-filter for larger sediments as well.

Water Filtration Reverse Osmosis (www.justinhealth.com/
reverse-osmosis) Here you can find an under-the-counter
reverse osmosis filter that Dr. J personally endorses.
Reverse osmosis has the highest level of filtration.

Water Pitcher Gravity Filter (www.justinhealth.com/water-
pitcher) Here is a more affordable water filter option,
especially if you can't modify the house you live in for a
water filter installation. This water pitcher filters out far
more toxins than your typical gravity water pitcher filter.

Micronutrients and Macronutrient Counter (www.
justinhealth.com/nutrient-counter) This is a nutrient
counter that will track your macronutrients like protein,
fat, carbs, and overall calories, which is standard. What
is different is that it will also look at micronutrients like
magnesium, potassium, etc.

Dexcom Blood Sugar Meter (www.justinhealth.com/dexcom)
This is a continuous blood glucose monitor; you may need
a doctor's prescription to access it.

FreeStyle Libre (www.justinhealth.com/libre) This is a
continuous blood glucose monitor; you may need a
doctor's prescription to access it.

KetoMojo Ketone and Blood Sugar Meter (www.justinhealth. com/ketomojo) This is an excellent blood sugar meter that will connect to your phone via Bluetooth and graph your blood sugar levels. It can also test for ketones.

Blue Blocking Glasses (www.justinhealth.com/glasses) These glasses are independently lab-tested to guarantee a blue light reduction of 99 percent or more.

Diet Reintroduction Handout (www.justinhealth.com/diet-reintroduction) This handout instructs you how to add foods back into your diet.

Recommended Products (www.justinhealth.com/approved-products) The list includes high-quality snacks, air filters, water filters, and devices that can improve your health.

Chapter 3

Thyroid Reboot Foundations Bundle (www.justinhealth. com/foundations) Here are several recommended thyroid supporting supplements mentioned in the book in easy-to-access bundles.

Digestive Support (www.justinhealth.com/digestive) These are some digestive-supporting supplements that Dr. J uses with his patients. Ranging from digestive acids, enzymes, bile support, and gut-healing nutrients.

Health Tracker (www.justinhealth.com/health-tracker) Here, you can efficiently manage and track your previous lab work. Additionally, there is an API feature that allows you to connect to your health insurance portal and upload PDFs of old lab tests. These documents will be automatically transcribed and uploaded to your portal, including graphed lab values, which will make it easier for you to assess your lab trends.

Comprehensive Stool Test (www.justinhealth.com/stool-test) This is a genetic stool test that Dr. J recommends that uses sensitive PCR DNA technology that will detect bacteria including H. pylori, parasites, and fungal overgrowth. This test also assesses gut inflammation, immune function, enzymes, and fat malabsorption.

SIBO Breath Test (www.justinhealth.com/breath-test) This is a lactulose breath test that will test for methane and hydrogen gas production to help assess small intestinal bacterial overgrowth.

Organic Acid Test OAT (www.justinhealth.com/organic-acid-test) This test looks at organic acids, giving us a window into the function of metabolic processes in the body like detoxification, mitochondrial function, nutritional deficiencies, gut bacteria, and fungal overgrowth.

Comprehensive Blood Test (www.justinhealth.com/comprehensive-blood-test) This is a comprehensive blood test that includes a CBC, metabolic panel, full thyroid panel, vitamin D panel, inflammation panel, and urinalysis.

Complete Thyroid Test (www.justinhealth.com/complete-thyroid-test) This is a comprehensive thyroid panel, including TSH, T4 free, T4 total, T3 free, T3 total, TPO ab, TG ab, and RT3.

Abridged Thyroid Test (www.justinhealth.com/abridged-thyroid-test) This is an abridged thyroid panel including TSH, T4 free, T3 free, TPO ab, and TG ab.

H. Pylori Breath Test (www.justinhealth.com/h-pylori-breath-test) This is a H. pylori breath test to help detect H. pylori.

Micronutrient Test (www.justinhealth.com/micro-nutrient-test) This is a test that will look at blood and urine to assess micronutrient levels.

Iron Test (www.justinhealth.com/iron-test) This is a comprehensive iron test looking at ferritin, iron saturation, IBC, iron total, and reticulocyte count.

Chapter 4

Thyroid Reboot Foundations Bundle (www.justinhealth.com/foundations) Here are several recommended thyroid supporting supplements mentioned in the book in easy-to-access bundles.

Urinary Adrenal Test (www.justinhealth.com/urine-adrenal-test) This is a comprehensive adrenal test that looks at free and total cortisol levels, cortisol rhythm throughout the day, and DHEA levels.

Urinary Complete Hormone Test (www.justinhealth.com/urine-complete-hormone-test) This is a comprehensive adrenal test that looks at free and total cortisol levels, cortisol rhythm throughout the day, and DHEA levels. It also looks at progesterone, estrone, estradiol, estriol, testosterone, androgen metabolites, estrogen detox pathways, and six organic acid tests.

Urine Sex Hormone Test (www.justinhealth.com/urine-sex-hormone-test) This test will look at progesterone, estrone, estradiol, estriol, testosterone, androgen metabolites, and estrogen detox pathways.

Adrenal Support (www.justinhealth.com/adrenal) These are some of the adrenal nutrients that Dr. J uses with his patients. Ranging from botanicals, nutrients, glandulars, and bio-identical hormones.

Adrenal Fatigue vs. Failure (www.justinhealth.com/adrenal-fatigue-vs-adrenal-failure) This blog post compares the misconceptions between adrenal fatigue or dysfunction and adrenal failure.

Cold Plunge (www.justinhealth.com/cold-plunge) Has many metabolic benefits to increase metabolism and supporting a health parasympathetic nervous system response.

Chapter 5

Thyroid Reboot Foundations Bundle (www.justinhealth.com/foundations) Here are several recommended thyroid supporting supplements mentioned in the book in easy-to-access bundles.

Diet Reintroduction Handout (www.justinhealth.com/diet-reintroduction) This handout will review the process by which Dr. J. recommends adding new foods to his patients' diets.

Genetic Gluten Test (www.justinhealth.com/gluten-testing) This is a genetic gluten test that will test HLA for celiac disease and can be used to detect gluten sensitivity. The markers include HLA-DQ2, (DQA1*05/DQB1*02), HLA-DQ8, HLA-DQA1*, and HLA-DQB1*.

Celiac Disease Panel (www.justinhealth.com/celiac-disease-panel) This is a comprehensive blood test looking at immunoglobulin A, interpretation, and tissue transglutaminase. These markers are used to diagnose celiac disease.

Food Allergy Panel (www.justinhealth.com/food-allergy-panel) This is a more comprehensive food allergy test, looking at markers beyond your typical IGE or even IGG immune reactions. We will look at other immune reactions, including T-cells.

Chapter 6

Thyroid Reboot Foundations Bundle (www.justinhealth.com/foundations) Here are several recommended thyroid supporting supplements mentioned in the book in easy-to-access bundles.

Detoxification Support (www.justinhealth.com/detox) These are some of the detoxification-supporting supplements Dr. J uses with his patients. Ranging from sulfur amino acids, glutathione, and liver tonifying herbs.

Infrared Sauna (www.justinhealth.com/sauna) Here you can find the specific sauna that Dr. J recommends to patients and that he personally uses.

Organic Pasture Fed Meats (www.justinhealth.com/meat) Here is a great site that sources grass-fed and organic food from Texas farms and can ship it anywhere in the USA.

Organic Acid Test OAT (www.justinhealth.com/organic-acid-test) This test looks at organic acids, giving us a window into the function of metabolic processes in the body like detoxification. It can also look at mitochondrial function, nutritional deficiencies, gut bacteria, and fungal overgrowth.

Urine Mold Testing (www.justinhealth.com/urine-mold-test) This test evaluates the mold toxins present in your urine. If your detox pathways are weak, using NAC or glutathione can help your body expel the mold toxins more effectively into the urine.

Environmental Mold Testing (www.justinhealth.com/environmental-mold-test) This is a mold plate test that can assess molds found in the environment, especially toxic molds that produce mycotoxins.

Environmental Mold Detox (www.justinhealth.com/environmental-mold-detox) This blend of botanicals can be used in a dry fogger as a safe way to help lower the mold in your environment.

Whole House Dehumidifier (wwww.justinhealth.com/dehumidifier) High humidity in your house can cause an elevation in mold. Decreasing your humidity with a dehumidifier can help decrease your mold levels.

Air Filtration (www.justinhealth.com/air-filters) Here is a high-quality air filter that Dr. J uses with his family and patients. This type of air filtration uses a HEPA air filter and an additional VOC filter that can filter other toxins typical air filters miss.

Heavy Metal Testing Urine (www.justinhealth.com/heavy-metal-test) This test looks for heavy metals in the urine. It is typically used with a chelation agent to provoke a detoxification response.

Comprehensive Blood Test (www.justinhealth.com/comprehensive-blood-test) This is a comprehensive blood test that includes a CBC, metabolic panel, full thyroid panel, vitamin D, inflammation, and urinalysis. The metabolic panel includes liver enzymes as well.

Whole House Filtration (www.justinhealth.com/water-filters) This is a recommendation for the whole-house filter Dr. J uses in his own home. This filter is carbon-based and has a pre- and post-filter for larger sediments as well.

Water Filtration Reverse Osmosis (www.justinhealth.com/reverse-osmosis) Here you can find an under-the-counter reverse osmosis filter that Dr. J personally endorses. Reverse osmosis has the highest level of filtration.

Sulfur Soap (www.justinhealth.com/soap) High quality 10 percent sulfur soap.

Chapter 7

Thyroid Reboot Foundations Bundle (www.justinhealth.com/foundations) Here are several recommended thyroid supporting supplements mentioned in the book in easy-to-access bundles.

GI Clearing Herbs (www.justinhealth.com/digestive) Here you can find some of the GI-clearing herbs that Dr. J uses with his patients. These clearing herbs range from GI Clear 1 through 6, and they contain some of the herbs mentioned in this chapter.

Comprehensive Stool Test (www.justinhealth.com/stool-test) This is a genetic stool test that Dr. J recommends that uses sensitive PCR DNA technology that will detect bacteria including H. pylori, parasites, and fungal overgrowth. This test also assesses gut inflammation, immune function, enzymes, and fat malabsorption.

Lyme & Coinfection Test (www.justinhealth.com/infection)
This test looks at Lyme disease-causing bacteria and ten
additional co-infectors. A positive result confirms DNA
presence, while a negative result doesn't rule out infection.
This urine-based test offers clearer insights into Lyme
disease and related infections.

Matula Tea (www.justinhealth.com/h.pylori-tea) Matula Tea is
an herbal blend originating from South Africa, traditionally
used for its potential health benefits, particularly in
promoting gastrointestinal health and as a natural remedy
to help eradicate *Helicobacter pylori* (*H. pylori*) infections.

Chapter 8

Thyroid Reboot Foundations Bundle (www.justinhealth.
com/foundations) Here are several recommended thyroid
supporting supplements mentioned in the book in easy-
to-access bundles.

Just In Health Supplements (www.justinhealth.com/
shop) You can find various supplements that Dr. J uses
personally as well as with his patients. They are organized
by categories for easy browsing.

Micronutrients Counter (www.justinhealth.com/nutrient-
counter) This is a nutrient counter that will track your
macronutrients like protein, fat, carbs, and overall calories,
which is standard. What is different is that it will also look
at micronutrients like magnesium, potassium, etc.

Organic Acid Test OAT (www.justinhealth.com/organic-acid-
test) This test looks at organic acids, giving us a window
into the function of metabolic processes in the body

like detoxification, mitochondrial function, nutritional deficiencies, gut bacteria, and fungal overgrowth.

Blood Test Review (www.justinhealth.com/blood-test-road-map) This is an Excel sheet that contains the reference range for thyroid labs as well as other tests Dr. J uses.

Urinary Iodine Test (www.justinhealth.com/iodine-test) This is a twenty-four-hour urinary test to assess iodine levels.

NutrEval Test (www.justinhealth.com/nutreval-test) is a comprehensive analysis that identifies nutritional deficiencies and imbalances in the body. By examining various biomarkers, it provides insights into one's metabolic health, including amino acid, fatty acid, and antioxidant levels.

Metabolomix+ Test (www.justinhealth.com/metabolimx-test) is a comprehensive assessment that evaluates an individual's metabolic health and function. By analyzing blood and urine, it provides insights into one's nutritional status, energy production, and detoxification processes.

Micronutrients Deficiency Test (www.justinhealth.com/micronutrient-deficiency-test) This test is an advanced diagnostic tool that uses lymphocyte stimulation to assess micronutrient levels and cellular function in the body. By evaluating vitamins, minerals, antioxidants, and other essential nutrients, it identifies deficiencies and imbalances.

Chapter 9

Access to Dr. J (www.justinhealth.com/free-consult) Here you can find virtual options to work with Dr. J if you want to dive in as a patient and get to the root of your thyroid and other health challenges.

Thyroid Reboot Foundations Bundle (www.justinhealth.com/foundations) Here are several recommended thyroid supporting supplements mentioned in the book in easy-to-access bundles.

Access to The Thyroid Course (www.justinhealth.com/thyroid-course) Here you can find Dr. J's course, which is an in-depth video version of this course in a live lecture format. There will be live Q&As to enhance your experience of the book.

Putting It Together (www.justinhealth.com/putting-it-together) How to put together an optimal functional medicine program It's important to address foundational issues while testing for root causes and stressors that are holding back your healing. Here is a podcast that will walk you through the right steps.

Find A Good Practitioner (www.justinhealth.com/find-a-practitioner) How to find a practitioner who has a comprehensive approach, addresses the root causes of health issues, and offers personalized treatment plans Consider compatibility in terms of communication and rapport, ensuring a strong patient-practitioner relationship for optimal health outcomes.

Health Tracker (www.justinhealth.com/health-tracker) Here you can manage and track your old lab work more efficiently.

Thyroid Reboot Recipes (www.justinhealth.com/thyroid-reboot-recipes) Dr. J's Thyroid Reboot Recipes will provide additional dietary advice and recipes to help supplement optimal thyroid health.